Table of Contents

Copyright and Limited Release

Disclaimers

Important Note to Reader

Chapter 1

INTRODUCTION

Free Bonus Downloads

Introduction

Active Patients and Shared Decision Making

Medical Errors

Evidence-Based Medicine

Health Information on the Internet

Book Organization and Scope

Chapter 2

BACKGROUND & DEFINITIONS

NCI Dictionary of Cancer Terms

NCI Drug Dictionary

NCI Thesaurus

NCI Metathesaurus

Controlled Vocabularies in Health

Medical Subject Headings (MeSH)

Burning Mouth Syndrome Journal Articles

Burning Mouth Syndrome Internet Articles and Research

Chapter 3

EPIDEMIOLOGY

Morbidity and Disease

Sources of Morbidity Statistics

Mortality and Disease

Sources of Mortality Statistics

Burning Mouth Syndrome Journal Articles

Burning Mouth Syndrome Internet Articles and Research

Chapter 4

RISK FACTORS & CAUSES

Risk Factors for Disease

Causes of Disease

Burning Mouth Syndrome Journal Articles

Burning Mouth Syndrome Internet Articles and Research

Chapter 5

SYMPTOMS & SIGNS

Distinguishing Symtoms from Signs

Types of Symptoms

Burning Mouth Syndrome Journal Articles

Burning Mouth Syndrome Internet Articles and Research

Chapter 6

DIAGNOSIS

The Diagnostic and Differential Diagnostic Process

Burning Mouth Syndrome Journal Articles

Burning Mouth Syndrome Internet Articles and Research

Chapter 7

PATHOPHYSIOLOGY

Understanding Pathophysiology

Burning Mouth Syndrome Journal Articles

Burning Mouth Syndrome Internet Articles and Research

Chapter 8

TREATMENT

Treatment and Therapy

Burning Mouth Syndrome Journal Articles

Burning Mouth Syndrome Internet Articles and Research

Chapter 9

PROGNOSIS

Defining Prognosis

Burning Mouth Syndrome Journal Articles

Burning Mouth Syndrome Internet Articles and Research

Chapter 10

APPLIED RESEARCH & RESOURCES

Alternative Health & Complementary Medicine

National Center for Complementary and Alternative Medicine (NCCAM)

Nutrition

National Institutes of Health Office of Dietary Supplements (ODS)

Biotechnology & Patents

Patent Information Online

Clinical Guidelines

Agency for Healthcare Research and Quality (AHRQ)

Drugs & Medications

Prescription and Over-the-Counter Drugs and Medications

Books

National Library of Medicine's Bookshelf

Journals

MEDLINE Journals - The Abridged Index Medicus (AIM)

All MEDLINE Journals

Current Journals

Current and Previously Indexed Journals

Using Filters to Search

Journal Articles

Types of Research Articles

The National Library of Medicine

National Library of Medicine Databases

MEDLINE

PubMed

PubMed Central

PubMed Journal Citations

PubMed Central (PMC) Journal Citations

FREE EBOOK DOWNLOADS

REFERENCES

Disclaimers

This publication is provided as a resource reference for patients, physicians, researchers, students, policymakers and any and all persons interested in finding the best research on health-related conditions. As a reference document, this publication provides an overview of, and links to historical and current developments in the understanding of specified illnesses and disease. Necessarily, this publication contains references to research conclusions that are both generally accepted and unconventional to the understanding and treatment of specified health conditions and disease. While every attempt has been made by the author and publisher to provide a comprehensive list of relevant resources and factual information pertaining to specific diseases and disorders, the author and publisher are not responsible for any omissions in research, or for the research conclusions or recommendations made by individuals referenced herein. As a result this publication should not be used to diagnosis or treat any health or medical condition without first consulting with a qualified health care professional. This publication is sold with the understanding that the author and publisher are not endorsing particular research conclusions or providing professional medical, legal, financial, or psychological advice and that the reader assumes all responsibility for the use of information contained herein.

Important Note to Reader

This book is one in a series of books on researching specific health conditions and disease.

The purpose of this series is twofold.

First, these books provide specific information on critical aspects of different diseases, disorders, and health conditions. The purpose of providing this information is to supply the reader with the most noteworthy, reliable, and important background on a variety of health conditions and concerns.

Second, these books provide a basic primer on researching health conditions and disease. This is accomplished by not only identifying the best available health and disease resources but also by teaching the reader the skills necessary to perform independent and thoughtful research to answer specific questions related to their unique health information needs.

As such, this book is both *informational* and *instructional*.

As an informational text, each book is totally unique and independent from any other book in this series. This is true because the resource information in each book is presented for a specific disease or health condition. Thus, each volume is unique from another based the particular characteristics of the health concern being discussed.

As a manual for instruction, each book in the series is similar, and in many places identical to the other books in the series in that each incorporates the same research principles, database sources, reference archives, and similar approaches to finding and utilizing the most reliable and current health information available today.

The dual nature of this book therefore begs the question:

"If I am interested in research about more than one disease or health condition should I purchase a separate volume for each disease?"

The honest answer is… "It depends."

If your primary purpose for reading for this book is the same as the primary reason this publication was written, that being to better understand a particular physical disease or psychological disorder then the answer is **"Yes,"** you should consider purchasing additional volumes as each book only provides factual information about the particular health condition or disease identified in the book title.

However, if you are purchasing this volume for bibliographic and reference information or to learn how to engage in professional-quality health care research by understanding what constitutes a reliable and current resource and research best practices, then the answer is a **"No,"** you should not purchase more than one volume in this series. This is because each volume will teach you the identical skills and empower you to research any disease or health condition on your own, therefore bypassing the need for the information resources found in the additional series volumes.

J.G.E.

CHAPTER 1

INTRODUCTION

Free Bonus Downloads

We have included **18 FREE** health and medical ebooks at the end of the book just for our readers. If you are reading this right now you belong to those who have access to these special free bonuses. Collectively, these ebooks constitute an entire health and medical library covering all types of disease and each aspect of health-related research.

Each ebook contains a detailed and fully functional Table of Contents to ensure you are able to simply and quickly navigate to your destination and access the precise information you need. Collectively, the ebooks include contributions from more than 1,000 of the most highly-esteemed medical, health, and research professionals. Since each is provided under either a Creative Commons or public domain license you are free to edit or adapt each book based on your individual needs.

The **FREE** ebooks included in your download bonus are:

- **The Encyclopedia of Disease** (14 volumes, 4,625 pages)
- **Dictionary of Clinical Research Terms** (268 pages)
- **Dictionary of Psychiatry Terminology** (167 pages)
- **The Complete Guide to Alternative and Complementary Medicine** (135 pages)
- **The Truth About Herbal Cures** (106 pages)

Each ebook is formatted to enable you to read your library anytime, anywhere in **all** of the formats listed below:

- **MOBI** - the standard format used by Amazon, allowing you to upload to your Kindle library and read on your Kindle e-reader or desktop, laptop, or mobile phone with the Kindle app)
- **AZW3** - the newer, more flexible format used by Amazon and available on the same devices as MOBI
- **EPUB** - the Nook, Kobo, and Apple format (iPod, iPhone, Apple computer) directly uploadable to each of these devices

- **PDF** - the traditional print- and computer-based document type, formatted to read exactly like a well-structured physical book.

Your ebook collection can be accessed using either one of the two links **found at the end of this book**. To ensure your privacy and security **NO** password or access code is required and **NO** cookies will be stored on your computer or other device.

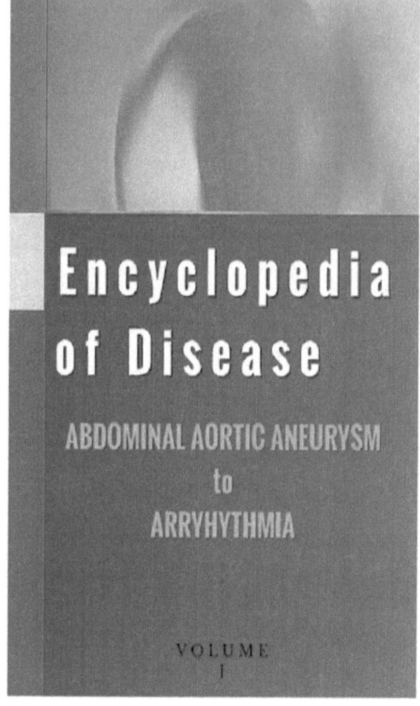

Encyclopedia of Disease (14 volumes, 4,625 pages *Volume I shown*)

DICTIONARY of CLINICAL RESEARCH TERMS

Second Edition

Walter McNulty, MD, MPH
Jennifer Rousset-Rowe, DO, MPH

Dictionary of Clinical Research Terms (268 pages)

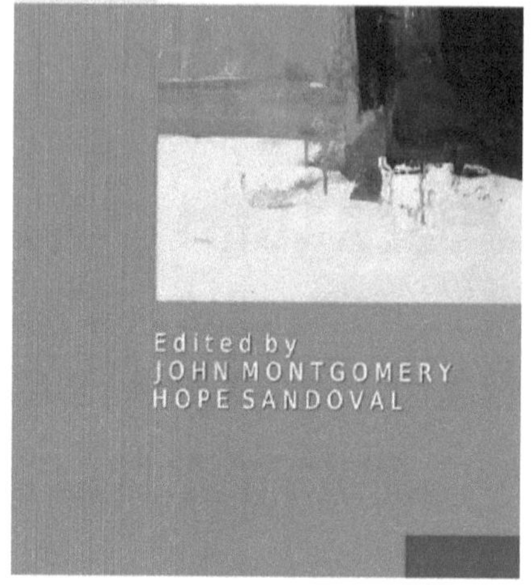

Dictionary of Psychiatry Terminology (167 pages)

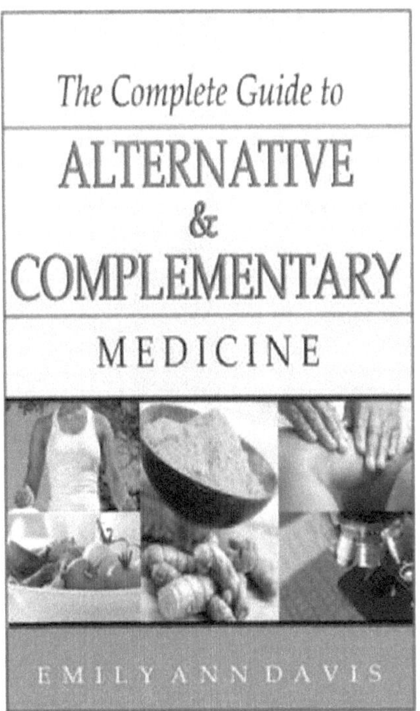

The Complete Guide to Alternative and Complementary Medicine (135 pages)

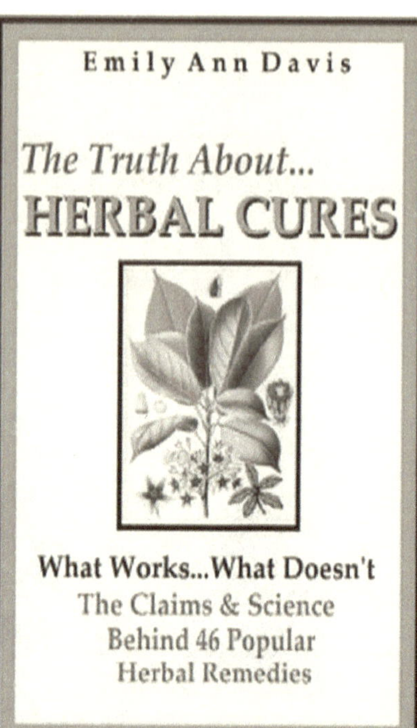

The Truth About Herbal Cures (106 pages)

Introduction

Broadly speaking, this book and the other volumes in this series are about health literacy. More specifically this book is about understanding the basic medical components and physiological nuance of your health condition (signs, symptoms, treatment, prognosis, etc.), researching and identifying the most authoritative and reliable information given your unique health needs (i.e. medical/physical/emotional circumstances), synthesizing this knowledge into a coherent whole, and applying your knowledge to your daily healthy living regime, or to the care of your patient or loved one.

Since this book is fundamentally about both the characteristics of Burning Mouth Syndrome and finding relevant information about this condition, it is ideal for both the patient and the student of medicine and the life sciences, as well as others in need of authoritative, valid, and sound health information. U.S. government health experts define health literacy as "the degree to which an individual has the capacity to obtain, communicate, process, and understand basic health information and services to make appropriate health decisions." Experts agree that more than half of the adult population in the U.S. can be termed "health illiterate" and that 9 out of 10 adults are unable to understand and correctly apply even the most basic health instructions recommended by a doctor or other health care professionals. The result is that 90 million Americans are unable to take even the most basic steps to prevent disease and manage their own health conditions. Sadly, the deficiency of health knowledge is not limited to the U.S., but is widespread worldwide. This lack of health literacy, or "health illiteracy," has serious consequences; including increases in preventable deaths, increases in personal health care costs, and poor health outcomes for a majority of adults and their children.

Active Patients and Shared Decision Making

Research has demonstrated that patients who take an active role in their medical care maintain more healthy lives, recover more quickly from illness and disease, and live longer. In addition to improving health outcomes, patients who actively participate in medical decision making report increased satisfaction with their treatment, their doctors, and the health care system in general. Research has further shown that more than half of all patients are dissatisfied with the role they play in making decisions about their own personal health care.

Rather than taking a passive or subordinate role in health care, active patients partner with doctors, nurses, specialists, and other health care professionals by assuming a leadership role in managing their personal health care. These patients schedule routine medical visits, follow through on doctor recommendations and, equally as important, stay informed about health trends and health conditions that impact them. By becoming educated, these patients take the personal responsibility to learn about disease and disorders, follow evidence-based medical guidelines communicated to them by health care professionals, and strive to become knowledgeable enough to find, understand, and follow the best and most current information about illness and chronic disease management.

Because of the overall benefits of active participation in health care decision making by patients, a new health care delivery paradigm known as Shared Decision Making, or SDM, is being advocated by hospitals, researchers, and patient advocacy groups worldwide. In study after study, research has consistently and conclusively demonstrated the effectiveness of this health care model in medical disciplines ranging from preventative care, to chronic disease management (such as diabetes), to pain management, and beyond. Moreover, studies have concluded that SDM is especially effective in combating the most deadly health conditions, including the screening and treatment of cancer and heart disease.

To become an active patient, it is critical that you first know where to find reliable health information and then understand how to apply this information to your own lifestyle, health conditions, and unique set of values and personal beliefs.

This, however, isn't always as simple as it sounds. Routinely, a patient's primary (if not only) resource for medical information is the World Wide Web. Unregulated and saturated with unscrupulous "charlatans," much of the health-related information on the Web is not only inaccurate but potentially dangerous and even life-threatening. Moreover, just as technological innovation has opened up Web publishing to anyone with a network connection and a little extra time, new self-publishing platforms are making it likewise as easy for these same people to publish important looking books, regardless of the author's credentials or expertise. It is for these reasons that this book has been written with one over-arching goal in mind, to give all patients the tools and resources to become "active" patients in the care and treatment of their particular disease, disorder, or other health condition.

However, becoming an active, informed patient is only half the equation. The other half involves holding health care professionals to this same high standard of knowledge. Today physicians, nurses, and other health care professionals face numerous challenges in keeping abreast of the latest research in illness and disease and current and appropriate clinical guidelines for delivering high quality health care to patients. Popular news is replete with stories of the "crisis" in health care caused by the diminishing number of medical students choosing careers in primary care and instead opting for more lucrative specializations such as orthopedic surgery, cardiology, gastroenterology, urology, dermatology, or radiology. The result is that fewer primary care physicians are seeing more patients, spending less time with each patient, and treating more ailments, all the while struggling to manage larger caseloads and having virtually no time to stay informed on the most critical research concerning the myriad of health conditions they treat on a daily basis.

Coupled with overburdened primary care physicians, health care delivery writ large has become increasingly fragmented and it is this fragmentation that has contributed to more and more medical errors as doctors fail to adequately diagnose and communicate life-threatening conditions to both patients and other members of the health care team responsible for patient care. In 1970, the American Board of Medical Specialties (ABMS) issued certificates in only 10 medical specialties and sub-specialties. Less than 20 years later this number increased to 66 and today approximately 145 medical specialties and sub-specialties are recognized by the ABMS. The consequence is that instead of seeing one or two doctors for a particular ailment, a patient may now see four or five different physicians and specialists to treat the same condition. While all this specialization can have a positive impact on patient health, this will only be true when each member of the health care team adequately and accurately communicates test results, patient observations, and other important medical information to all the other members of the team. When communication is lacking and information is not made available to the entire team, the consequences to the patient can be catastrophic, or even life-threatening in some instances.

Finally, in America the recent expansion of the number of persons seeking and receiving health care as a result of the Affordable Care Act (ACA or

"Obamacare") has overwhelmed a system already bursting at its resource seams, resulting in still more patients seeking more care from the already stressed health care system. For many of the more than eight (8) million new ACA patients, this is the first time in their lives they have had access to routine health care, including periodic check-ups, preventative care, and other basic health services. Due to the poor health care histories for these individuals and in contrast to the average patient in the pre-ACA health care population, this new group of patients is likely to enter the system with more chronic health conditions like diabetes, obesity, and high blood pressure (conditions that could have been prevented if they only had access to health care earlier). Therefore, while the ACA has increased the number of new patients by only about 3%, from approximately 256 million patients to 264 million patients, per capita it is anticipated that these patients will require more health care services than the existing patient population.

Given our beleaguered and disjointed health care system, it is no wonder that physicians and other health care professionals have virtually no time and even less energy to adequately stay informed on the most recent developments in their field. Furthermore, the sheer amount of new health information available today is immense, doubling in volume once every five (5) years. Advances in science (most notably in the study of human DNA and progress made in identifying and mapping all genes in the human genome) and technology (such as the ability to manipulate massive amounts of study data in near real-time) has rapidly increased the rate of medical advancement and made seemingly new medical innovations quickly obsolete. The cumulative effect is some doctors basing important medical decisions on outdated medical guidelines and best practices.

Because of the current state of affairs, this book is also for the health care professional. Using the same resources for patients and health professionals the goal of this book is twofold. First, this book will identify the best books, journals, journal articles, and Web resources about Burning Mouth Syndrome available to the patient and the health care provider, therefore giving the reader a quick inventory of current research and a convenient reference during times when performing firsthand research is simply not practical, such as during a patient's appointment with her doctor. Second, it explains the most basic "mechanics" of health research and how to find and use the most trustworthy and comprehensive health care journals, databases, books, and electronic resources available in the world today. In this regard, the author hopes that this book empowers both the patient and health care professional by making each a more informed, educated, and responsible user of timely and cutting edge health information.

Though not its primary purpose, this book is in some respects a do-it-yourself guide to health-related research and resources and, as such, it is important to note this book is not prescriptive; meaning that while this book does identify limited information about causes or risk factors of Burning Mouth Syndrome, recommend diagnostic or treatment procedures, etc., this is NOT the primary purpose of this book. Instead, this book should be used as a tool for the reader to explore and find information about Burning Mouth Syndrome on her or his own based on their specific circumstances as patient, loved one, health care professional, researcher, or public policy-maker; keeping foremost in mind the needs and value-systems of the patient. Since health information is constantly updated and rapid medical innovation the rule rather than the exception, the author hopes this volume is not used once and forgotten to collect dust on the bookshelf, but continually and routinely referred to in order to stay abreast on the latest medical developments and apply the most recent best practices over the long-term.

Further, for patients or other "lay-persons" using this reference it is vital to understand that the knowledge gained by applying the recommendations and practices found in this book do not replace the advice and recommendations of your physician. Instead, in the spirit of SDM, the research gathered from methods used in this book should be shared with your physician and health care team to collectively determine the best course of action for a health condition keeping foremost in your specific circumstances and needs.

Finally, the author recognizes that the value of this book is based less on its content and more on its application to real-world health questions. It is therefore expected that a patient or a patient's loved one will find different utility in its pages than a health care professional. For the former, it is the author's hope that this book reduces the mystery surrounding scientific medical research and empowers the patient through knowledge and confident health care decision making. For the latter, and particularly the more highly educated health care professional, some of this material may be remedial and some simply a refresher of things you once knew but have forgotten. Since this book has also been written for the student researcher, it is the hope that this edition proves to be a valuable introduction to researching Burning

Mouth Syndrome and studying disease and health conditions in general.

Medical Errors

If you're a patient or have a loved-one receiving medical treatment and are still not convinced about the importance about being active in your health care treatment consider a 2013 article entitled *A New, Evidence-based Estimate of Patient Harms Associated with Hospital Care*, authored by John T. James, PhD, and published in the well-regarded Journal of Patient Safety. In this research article Dr. James estimates that between 210,000 and 440,000 patients die each year from preventable medical errors. If these estimates are accurate, then medical errors are the third leading cause of death in America, behind only heart disease and cancer. Similarly, other health care data suggests that 17% of all deaths in America each year can attributed to medical errors. What's as disturbing, is that these estimates only include medical errors resulting in death and do not include other harmful consequences of preventable medical errors; including permanent physical or biological damage to the patient, longer periods of hospitalization, and a lower overall quality of life. Many experts agree that if these secondary consequences of medical errors were considered the true devastation caused by medical errors would be significantly higher.

Reinforcing James' findings, another report, this one by the Office of the Inspector General for Department of Health and Human Services, studied patient care for individuals on Medicare. This 2010 study concluded that 180,000 **Medicare-only** patients die each year as a result of poor hospital care.

In his study, Dr. James cites five (5) types of preventable medical errors: errors of commission, errors of omission, errors of communication, errors of context, and diagnostic errors. **Errors of commission** occur when a health professional administers a procedure that was either performed improperly or should not have been performed at all. On the other hand **errors of omission** simply means that, based on the best medical evidence, a procedure that should have been administered, wasn't performed at all. **Communication errors** occur between two or more health professionals or between health professionals and a patient and, as the name implies, happen when critical information is not shared with members of the health care team or the patient. Communication errors can lead to a misunderstanding by medical staff as to the correct patient diagnosis or prescribed treatment regime or cause a patient to unintentionally engage in activities that are contrary to acceptable established medical recommendations for their particular disease or disorder. Similarly, **errors of context** occur when a health professional fails to consider the unique circumstances of a patient in their "post-discharge" treatment. The example used by James is the patient who lacks the mental capacity to follow an ongoing, complex treatment plan or the patient who does not have access to follow-up medical care due to financial or geographical restrictions. Finally, **diagnostic errors** occur when the incorrect diagnosis is given to a patient. Diagnosis errors often result in inappropriate treatment, ineffective treatment, and a delay in the administration of the correct treatment.

Given the troubling prevalence of medical errors, it is obvious that current diagnostic and treatment shortcomings in our health care delivery system have very real, frequently deadly implications, for the unenlightened patient and the ill-informed health care professional. Thus, it is no exaggeration to strongly caution the uninformed, un-involved patient to proceed at her own risk.

Evidence-Based Medicine

Evidence-based medicine is currently the most widely accepted and applied model of patient care in Western medicine. The most commonly accepted definition of evidence-based (EBM) medicine is one offered by Dr. David Sackett who defines EBM as "the conscientious, explicit and judicious use of current best evidence in making decisions about the care of the individual patient. It means integrating individual clinical expertise with the best available external clinical evidence from systematic research."(Sackett, Rosenberg, Gray, Haynes, & Richardson, 1996).

Therefore, EBM is the integration of the best medical evidence, as found through literature reviews and research, the clinical expertise and experience of the doctor, and a constant recognition of patient values and concerns. Fundamental to the EBM model is its reliance on research and literature reviews to give the doctor and patient the best possible benchmark or baseline information to begin to answer relevant clinical questions and formulate a treatment plan both appropriate and acceptable to the patient. It is the goal of this book to provide the reader with both the basic medical literature research tools, as well as a bibliography of some of the important research itself. However, it is important to remember that even though evidence and research are primary in the EBM decision making process, it is not the sole deciding factor in determining patient care and on a case-by-case basis may in some instances not even be the most important consideration.

The EBM process begins by identifying a clinical problem and then applying this problem to a specific question about treating and caring for the individual patient. Based on the question, the doctor or researcher then determines the best available resource or resources to answer that question. Next, the literature is reviewed keeping in mind two important questions. First, is the literature **valid**, meaning does it accurately represent the truth as we know it today and does it have a sound basis in reason and fact. Second, does the literature offer advice and recommendations that are **applicable** to the patient and therefore will, if followed, offer a reasonable expectation of a successful patient outcome. Once the doctor has made her evaluation and formed a recommendation or alternative recommendations, she presents her conclusions and recommendations to the patient and in consult together they examine the evidence and discuss the patient's preferences and values to agree on a course of medical treatment.

Health Information on the Internet

Since most disease and health-related information is accessed by both patients and medical professionals via the Internet, either through general queries using search engines like Google or by directly accessing professional databases and information repositories, it is important be able to determine what constitutes quality health information. A 2013 survey by the Pew Research Center found that "59% of U.S. adults have looked online for information about a range of health related topics in the past year", and "35% of U.S. adults say they have gone online specifically to try to figure out what medical condition they or someone else might have." While the Internet can be a quality resource to find information quickly and easily, there are many important questions to answer to evaluate the information you find online, such as:

Which websites and databases are most reliable?

How do you analyze the information you've found?

How current is the information you've found?

Unfortunately, not everyone reading this book is a medical professional and everyone doesn't possess the same background or knowledge base to understand and filter all the information found online. This section will therefore examine some factors to consider when evaluating health information on the Internet.

More often than not, your first foray into researching all but the most basic health information online will end in confusion. While there is no shortage of health information on the Internet, at best much of what you will find will consist of over-generalizations of complex conditions, and analysis and recommendations not tailored to your specific concerns. At worst some of the information you find online will be founded upon baseless scientific conclusions, and downright dangerous home remedies. Certainly, your first rule of thumb needs to be that under no circumstance should you trust the veracity of everything written online. To make sense of what you find it is critical to keep a number of questions in mind prior to acting on any online health advice:

First, consider the source.

Look for an "about us" page. What is the original source of the information and what are the credentials of the person or organization that provided it? This information could be very telling.

Notice whether or not the website providing health related information shares its source(s)? If it does, is it a reliable source? Remember, much (if not most) information posted on websites actually originates from a third-party source. If the organization or person that owns or administers the website did not author the content the actual source should be conspicuously identified. Also, if the information wasn't written by a medical expert, was the information reviewed and approved for quality by an expert with professional credentials in that field?

If a non-medical person or organization wrote the article is it reliable? You should limit your research to only reliable sources. A reliable source could include websites published published by the U.S. government, non-for-profit entities, and universities or other institutions of higher learning. Respectively, these websites can be identified with dot gov, dot org or dot edu URL extensions. Does information on the website appear to be more opinion than fact? If it is opinion-based, does it come from a an expert area of study or unbiased and objective organization such as a medical association or research institute? These sites are generally the most trustworty as they are not affiliated with insurance or pharmaceutical companies, and therefore have no profit-based motive (or appearance of one) in providing certain conclusions or advice. Having said that, it is still recommended you to dig deeper to discover exactly where the information originated.

Today, most web search engines like Google make it easy to limit your searches to .org or .gov websites. Simply type in your search term (enclosed in quotations for multiple words) followed by "site:.org" or "site:.gov" without the quotations here of course. Always remember to include the dot after the colon in "site."

For example, to search the broad topic of Burning Mouth Syndrome simply type:

"Burning Mouth Syndrome" site:.org

or

"Burning Mouth Syndrome" site:.gov

Domain names with the .com web extension generally represent businesses or other for profit companies. Business websites have the primary purpose of selling products or services, instead of providing reliable health information. If this is the case, the health information could be skewed to make their product or service more appealing.

While commercial sites **may** offer some useful and accurate information you will want to remain vigilant and be sure to cross-check any of the information you find with a more reliable source. While it is possible that the information can be trusted, if it seems to be provided only to make a certain product or service more appealing it is best to be skeptical and move on to the next resource.

Finally, a third source of online information is websites published by individuals. Many of these sites offer support and advice about coping with certain conditions and their treatments. While these websites can contain reliable and useful information, it is necessarily biased by only one person's experience. Additionally, diseases and health conditions impact different people differently and there are numerous factors that need to be considered before relying wholesale on one person's experience. These factors may be demographic, such as age or gender, physical, including the person's overall health or other aggravating health conditions, or even the quality of health care the individual received.

Second, how current is the information?

Rapid advances in research means health information is continually changing. Daily, research discoveries and advancements change the landscapes in our understanding of countless diseases. As such, it is critical that a website clearly idenifies the date it was last updated. Most reliable web pages will include information about when the information was last updated or reviewed, in addition to a statement about how information is reviewed to stay current. The date is usually located towards the end of an article. If no date is posted, located the copyright notice. This will tell you the date the article was originally published or written and the publishing organization, if applicable. If the article is more than a year or two old, you are likely better off finding more current information.

Third, does the site present facts and not opinion?

Information should be clearly written, based in fact and present the full scope of the issue being studied, and not just selective anecdotes. The content should be easily verified from a trustworthy information source such as professional journal articles, abstracts, or doctors and other medical professionals.

Fourth, who is the intended audience?

It should be clearly stated on the website whether the information is intended for the consumer, or the health professional. Many websites have separate web pages for patients and doctors or health care professionals. Be sure to use the information that is most relevant to your information needs.

Fifth, be skeptical.

Claims that sound too good to be true often are. Your goal should be to find current, unbiased information based on scientifically valid research. If you're a patient, it is important to remember that no matter how confident you are in your online research it can not replace the advice of your doctor, as she is most familiar with your specific medical circumstances. Your doctor is the best person to answer questions about your personal health. She not only understands your health history and any medication you take, she also understands the plethora of other health factors that may be involved and interact and she's committed to providing the best possible care and treatment.

Book Organization and Scope

This book begins by providing the reader with background information and definitions related to Burning Mouth Syndrome. Importantly, the second chapter also identifies and explains specific high-quality resources the reader can trust when performing individual health research on specific topics and sub-topics. Chapters 3 through 9 proceed to discuss the individual components of *all* health-related conditions, including epidemiology, risk factors and cause, signs and symptoms, diagnosis, pathophysiology, treatment, and prognosis. Importantly, each of these chapters begin by explaining precisely what is a meant by a doctor when she discusses each of these concepts and ends with an examination of how each applies to the medical condition of Burning Mouth Syndrome. While this book focuses on the "nut-and-bolts" of Burning Mouth Syndrome, Chapter 10 concludes by providing the the interested reader with additional resources to expand their research to other areas, including but not limited to the role nutrition in preventing or treating Burning Mouth Syndrome, alternative therapies, and biotechnology.

Importantly, as a research reference, throughout this book hundreds of articles are identified to enable the reader examine particular issues in depth. Each list of references contains a wide assortment of articles and includes research studies and articles geared towards readers of all levels of sophistication, from research novices and patients to and medical and health-care professionals. Each article is hyperlinked directly to the source allowing the reader to access without leaving the book. Additionally, each reference is linked directly and not hidden beneath confusing anchor text thereby allowing the reader to identify the precise source and location of the article for further future reference.

While this book is organized in a manner that most closely resembles the order of disease or disorder progression, from pre-disability considerations to symptoms, treatment, and eventual outcome, it is first and foremost a reference book. This means a reader can read chapters and sections in isolation and without first reading a preceding chapter or section, as the entire book is written in a manner making it easy for the reader to refer to areas of immediate interest without fear of losing meaning or nuance that may have been discussed earlier in the book.

CHAPTER 2

BACKGROUND

&

DEFINITIONS

The purpose of this chapter is to provide the reader with resources to find high-level definitions of terminology associated with Burning Mouth Syndrome. The easiest way to begin your understanding of complex health concepts is to first understand the definitions of key words and phrases commonly associated with a disease or illness. It is helpful to look up the words you are unfamiliar with, and keep a list of definitions for your reference. Often, a common term in a non-scientific context has a completely different meaning than the same term has in medicine, so be prepared to investigate and find words that are more familiar to you if you cannot understand a term or make the standard definition work in your particular context. As you become more familiar with your topic, the vocabulary will become less daunting and difficult ideas will be more understandable. Once you have a grasp of the content of your research, spend some time thinking about the research. Critically interpret what the results mean and how they are relevant to the disease. Keep in mind that in contrast to words used in everyday writing or conversation, scientific and medical terms have very precise meanings. In this regard, you will frequently encounter two or more medical terms that *seem* to have identical meanings, only to discover later that the distinction between these terms is critically important in a medical context.

This chapter will first identify the best sources for finding reliable definitions and explanations for complex health and medical terms and introduce the concept of a "controlled vocabularly." This chapter will conclude with definitions of the most commonly used terms associated with Burning Mouth Syndrome.

NCI Dictionary of Cancer Terms

The *National Cancer Institute (NCI) Dictionary of Cancer Terms* contains definition and information for 7,665 medical terms. While developed and hosted by the NCI, the dictionary contains definitions for both cancer- and non-cancer-related medical concepts. To search, simply type in your search term and click the **go** button. To find all words in the dictionary that include your search term, click the radio button **Contains** and all definitions with your search term will be available. For example, searching the term "thyroid" will return results for 28 terms containing the word "thyroid" including "anaplastic thyroid cancer" "autoimmune thyroiditis," "familial isolated hyperparathyroidism," etc. You can also select the letter your term begins with and scroll to the term you are looking up. The search box contains an **autosuggest** feature so after you type in the first three letters of the word, you will be presented with the first 10 terms that begin with those letters. If your word doesn't appear within the first 10 suggestions simply continue to type in additional letters and eventually the dictionary will narrow its suggestions to the term you need. This is particularly helpful for longer terms and words difficult to spell. If you want to turn the autosuggest feature off simply hit escape or click **close** within the autosuggest box. The results include the definition for your selected terms as well as a pronunciation guide. If you want to hear how the word sounds, simply click the audio radio icon button next to the term name. The NCI Dictionary of Cancer Terms can be accessed at: http://www.cancer.gov/dictionary

NCI Drug Dictionary

The NCI Drug Dictionary defines terms and alternative research links for medications and drug agents used for cancer theryapy, as well as countless other health conditions. The search engine operates in a manner identical to the one used by the NCI Dictionary of Cancer Terms so the same tips apply. All definitions include synonyms and generic and brand names for the drug. One excellent feature of the the NCI Drug Dictionary is that it also includes links to both open and closed clinical research trials related to that medication. The NCI Drug Dictionary can be found at: http://www.cancer.gov/drugdictionary

NCI Thesaurus

The NCI Thesaurus (NCIt) is a database of reference terms for many health-related from the NCI and other health databases.

The NCIt is updated frequently by a team of medical experts and contains more than 200,000 links and cross-references to other research information related to your term. Most people believe that a thesaurus is used only to identify synonyms for individual words or phrases. This is not totally correct as the more important purpose of a good thesaurus is to identify related concepts and ideas. In this regard the NCI Thesaurus and the NCI Metathesaurus (discussed below) are wonderful resources to reference when defining terms and determining the scope of your information needs.

The thesaurus can be searched at: http://ncit.nci.nih.gov.

If you prefer to work offline, the entire thesaurus can also be downloaded at: http://evs.nci.nih.gov/ftp1/NCI_Thesaurus.

NCI Metathesaurus

The NCI Metathesaurus (NCIm) is a vast medical research terminology database that provides definition and conceptual information for more than 4 million terms related to clinical care, biomedical research, and health care administration in general. The NCIm also has more than 22 million links and cross-references to additional concepts and information related to health and disease. To search the NCIm simply go to: http://ncim.nci.nih.gov/ncimbrowser.

Controlled Vocabularies in Health

The single most important purpose of a controlled vocabulary is to make searching a database easier. The Library Archives of Canada defines a controlled vocabulary as an "established list of standardized terminology for use in indexing and retrieval of information." Controlled vocabularies are used to capture, store, organize, search, analyze, and normalize information allowing for the exchange of information across different platforms.

While the term controlled vocabulary may seem foreign, you are likely already familiar with applications of the concept of in other contexts. Using a series of cross-references, the Yellow Page listings in a telephone book use a controlled vocabulary to make searching for specific types of businesses or organizations easier. For example, a Yellow Page search for "Doctors" doesn't list doctors at all but instead says "*see* Chiropractors; Physicians - MD & DO; Podiatrists; Psychologists" thereby directing the reader to search for a doctor or type of doctor under these headings instead. This alternative listing for "Doctors" is a controlled vocabulary and like all controlled vocabularies serves three very important purposes.

The first is to keep the size of a database manageable. Imagine the amount of needless repetition that would occur if under the heading "Doctors" a complete listing of doctors was shown and the identical list appeared again under the subject heading "Physicians - MD & DO." Consider then the additional clutter created for duplicate listings for "Cars" and "Automobiles," "Grocery" and "Supermarkets," "Churches" and "Worship Services," "Job Services," and "Employment" and on and on. If this were done, it wouldn't take long for the size of the Yellow Pages in even communities of modest size to exceed that of a complete set of the old Encyclopedia Britannica. This concept of managing the size of information also holds true for computerized databases where the space needed to store duplicate entries is prohibitive in terms of bandwidth and storage costs.

The second, and more important purpose of the controlled vocabulary, is to make your search more efficient and more precise. Using our Yellow Pages example, imagine if a search under the term "Doctor" yielded nothing and the term itself wasn't even listed and you were expected to know to look under "Physicians - MD & DO" instead. While many people may have the wherewithal to look to the "Physician" listing this may not be true for people looking for contact information for businesses or organization in more esoteric fields. Thus, the controlled vocabulary makes it easy to find what you need by essentially saying "you're close, good try but go here instead and you will find exactly what you need."

Finally, controlled vocabularies make complex topics like medicine accessible to novices and other non-subject-matter-expert researchers. Have you ever had a rough concept of what you were you trying to locate but either didn't know its precise term or were unable to recall it? In instances like this a controlled vocabulary can be indispensable allowing you to enter a term close to the one needed but not exact and then returning a list of related concepts and terms where one is likely to meet your precise needs. In this way, a controlled vocabulary acts like a thesaurus of words or phrases. While some believe a thesaurus returns a list of exact synonyms for a chosen word, in truth the meanings for words in a thesaurus are most often similar but not exact. Therefore, when searching a thesaurus you really aren't trying to find a *fancier* word with the same meaning but a word that most precisely communicates the the idea you are attempting to convey in terms of meaning, magnitude, or degree.

In the online world, most websites and databases that store large sets of information incorporate at least a basic form controlled vocabularies. If you are familiar with the online concept of "keyword tagging" (like the use of the hash tag "#" in twitter "tweets" to affiliate messages with other message on the same topic), this is exactly what controlled vocabularies attempt to accomplish, albeit in a more sophisticated and organized manner. Like keyword tagging, establishing a controlled vocabulary is not a one-time endeavor, but a constant and ongoing exercise where categories and search words and phrases are updated continuously to accommodate new terms, ideas, and discoveries.

In the age of technology, it is important to point out that contrary to our Yellow Pages example the use of controlled vocabulary today is almost exclusively the province of the Internet. In Health and Medicine, the international gold standard of controlled vocabularies is known as MeSH, or Medical Subject Headings. MeSH is discussed further below.

Medical Subject Headings (MeSH)

MeSH or Medical Subject Headings is the U.S. National Library of Medicine's thesaurus. Use MeSH as a starting point for your research to collect relevant keywords and terms for further searches in the databases discussed later in this book. Since MeSH is both a controlled vocabulary and thesaurus the terms that appear in a MeSH search also include term definitions. These definitions should be recorded together with the MeSH search terms. Use MeSH definitions to understand important concepts and MeSH terms to establish a list of keywords for more in-depth and precise research.

MeSH is used by the NLM to catalogue all MEDLINE and PubMED databases, as well as NLM database of documents, books, and video and other NLM holdings. MeSH can be accessed by going to http://www.ncbi.nlm.nih.gov/mesh.

Burning Mouth Syndrome Journal Articles

Al Quran, F. A. M. (2004). Psychological profile in burning mouth syndrome. *Oral Surgery, Oral Medicine, Oral Pathology, Oral Radiology, and Endodontics, 97*(3), 339–344. http://doi.org/10.1016/j.tripleo.2003.09.017

Balasubramaniam, R., Klasser, G. D., & Delcanho, R. (2009). Separating oral burning from burning mouth syndrome: Unravelling a diagnostic enigma. *Australian Dental Journal.* http://doi.org/10.1111/j.1834-7819.2009.01153.x

Barker, K. E., & Savage, N. W. (2005). Burning mouth syndrome: An update on recent findings. *Australian Dental Journal.* http://doi.org/10.1111/j.1834-7819.2005.tb00363.x

Boy-Metin, Z., Kayhan, K. B., & Unür, M. (2008). Burning mouth syndrome. *Kulak Burun Boğaz Ihtisas Dergisi : KBB = Journal of Ear, Nose, and Throat, 18*(3), 188–96. Retrieved from http://www.ncbi.nlm.nih.gov/pubmed/19388467

Brufau-Redondo, C., Martín-Brufau, R., Corbalán-Velez, R., & De Concepción-Salesa, a. (2002). Burning mouth syndrome. *British Dental Journal, 45*(6), 237–241. http://doi.org/10.1111/j.1526-4637.2010.01035.x

Brufau-Redondo, C., Martin-Brufau, R., Corbalan-Velez, R., & de Concepcion-Salesa, A. (2008). {[}Burning mouth syndrome{]}. *Actas Dermosifiliogr, 99*(6), 431–440.

Cerchiari, D. P., de Moricz, R. D., Sanjar, F. A., Rapoport, P. B., Moretti, G., & Guerra, M. M. (2006). Burning mouth syndrome: etiology. *Brazilian Journal of Otorhinolaryngology, 72*(3), 419–23. http://doi.org/S0034-72992006000300021 [pii]

Cibirka, R. M., Nelson, S. K., & Lefebvre, C. A. (1999). A review of burning mouth syndrome. *The Journal of Prosthetic Dentistry, 78*(1), 29–35.

Coon, E. A., & Laughlin, R. S. (2012). Burning mouth syndrome in Parkinson's disease: Dopamine as cure or cause? *Journal of Headache and Pain, 13*(3), 255–257. http://doi.org/10.1007/s10194-012-0421-1

Crow, H. C., & Gonzalez, Y. (2012). Burning Mouth Syndrome. *Oral and Maxillofacial Surgery Clinics of North America, 65*(5), 343–347. http://doi.org/10.4248/IJOS10008

Crow, H. C., & Gonzalez, Y. (2013). Burning Mouth Syndrome. *Oral and*

Maxillofacial Surgery Clinics of North America.
http://doi.org/10.1016/j.coms.2012.11.001

Fedele, S., Fricchione, G., Porter, & Mignogna, M. (2007a). Stomatodynia or burning mouth syndrome. *Acta Dermatovenerologica Croatica ADC Hrvatsko Dermatolosko Drustvo, 100*(4), 231–235. Retrieved from http://discovery.ucl.ac.uk/148057/

Fedele, S., Fricchione, G., Porter, S. R., & Mignogna, M. D. (2007b). Stomatodynia or burning mouth syndrome. *Acta Dermatovenerologica Croatica ADC Hrvatsko Dermatolosko Drustvo, 11*(4), 231–235. Retrieved from http://discovery.ucl.ac.uk/148057/

Forssell, H., Teerijoki-Oksa, T., Kotiranta, U., Kantola, R., Bäck, M., Vuorjoki-Ranta, T.-R., … Estlander, A.-M. (2012). Pain and pain behavior in burning mouth syndrome: a pain diary study. *Journal of Orofacial Pain, 26*(2), 117–25. Retrieved from http://www.ncbi.nlm.nih.gov/pubmed/22558611

Friedman, D. I. (2010). Topirimate-induced burning mouth syndrome. *Headache, 50*(8), 1383–1385. http://doi.org/10.1111/j.1526-4610.2010.01720.x

Grushka, M., Epstein, J. B., & Gorsky, M. (2002). Burning mouth syndrome. *American Family Physician, 65*(4). http://doi.org/10.3748/wjg.v19.i5.665

Grushka, M., Epstein, J. B., & Gorsky, M. (2002). Burning mouth syndrome. *Am Fam Physician, 65*(4), 615–620. Retrieved from http://www.ncbi.nlm.nih.gov/entrez/query.fcgi?cmd=Retrieve&db=PubMed&dopt=Citation&list_uids=11871678

Gurvits, G. E., & Tan, A. (2013). Burning mouth syndrome. *World Journal of Gastroenterology : WJG, 19*(5), 665–72. http://doi.org/10.3748/wjg.v19.i5.665

Hagelberg, N., Forssell, H., Rinne, J. O., Scheinin, H., Taiminen, T., Aalto, S., … Jääskeläinen, S. (2003). Striatal dopamine D1 and D2 receptors in burning mouth syndrome. *Pain, 101*(1-2), 149–154. http://doi.org/10.1016/S0304-3959(02)00323-8

Huang, W., Rothe, M. J., & Grant-Kels, J. M. (1996). The burning mouth syndrome. *Journal of the American Academy of Dermatology, 34*(1), 91–98. http://doi.org/10.1016/S0190-9622(96)90840-3

Jääskeläinen, S. K. (2012). Pathophysiology of primary burning mouth syndrome. *Clinical Neurophysiology*. http://doi.org/10.1016/j.clinph.2011.07.054

Klasser, G. D., Epstein, J. B., & Villines, D. (2011). Management of burning mouth syndrome. *Journal (Canadian Dental Association)*, *77*, b151. Retrieved from http://www.ncbi.nlm.nih.gov/pubmed/22260804

Klasser, G. D., Fischer, D. J., & Epstein, J. B. (2008). Burning Mouth Syndrome: Recognition, Understanding, and Management. *Oral and Maxillofacial Surgery Clinics of North America*. http://doi.org/10.1016/j.coms.2007.12.012

Koszewicz, M., Mendak, M., Konopka, T., Koziorowska-Gawron, E., & Budrewicz, S. (2012). The characteristics of autonomic nervous system disorders in burning mouth syndrome and Parkinson disease. *Journal of Orofacial Pain*, *26*(4), 315–20. Retrieved from http://www.ncbi.nlm.nih.gov/pubmed/23110271

Lamey, P. J., & Lamb, A. B. (1994). Lip component of burning mouth syndrome. *Oral Surgery, Oral Medicine, and Oral Pathology*, *78*(5), 590–593. http://doi.org/10.1016/0030-4220(94)90169-4

Lauria, G., Majorana, A., Borgna, M., Lombardi, R., Penza, P., Padovani, A., & Sapelli, P. (2005). Trigeminal small-fiber sensory neuropathy causes burning mouth syndrome. *Pain*, *115*(3), 332–337. http://doi.org/10.1016/j.pain.2005.03.028

López-Jornet, P., Camacho-Alonso, F., & Andujar-Mateos, P. (2011). A prospective, randomized study on the efficacy of tongue protector in patients with burning mouth syndrome. *Oral Diseases*, *17*(3), 277–282. http://doi.org/10.1111/j.1601-0825.2010.01737.x

López-Jornet, P., Camacho-Alonso, F., Andujar-Mateos, P., Sánchez-Siles, M., & Gómez-Garcia, F. (2010). Burning mouth syndrome: an update. *Medicina Oral, Patología Oral Y Cirugía Bucal*, *15*(4), e562–8. Retrieved from http://www.ncbi.nlm.nih.gov/pubmed/23772971

Marino, R., Capaccio, P., Pignataro, L., & Spadari, F. (2009). Burning mouth syndrome: The role of contact hypersensitivity. *Oral Diseases*, *15*(4), 255–258. http://doi.org/10.1111/j.1601-0825.2009.01515.x

Marino, R., Torretta, S., Capaccio, P., Pignataro, L., & Spadari, F. (2010). Different therapeutic strategies for burning mouth syndrome: preliminary data. *Journal of Oral Pathology & Medicine : Official Publication of the International Association of Oral Pathologists and the American Academy of Oral Pathology, 39*(8), 611–616. http://doi.org/10.1111/j.1600-0714.2010.00922.x

Mignogna, M. D., Adamo, D., Schiavone, V., Ravel, M. G., & Fortuna, G. (2011). Burning Mouth Syndrome Responsive to Duloxetine: A Case Report. *Pain Medicine, 12*(3), 466–469. http://doi.org/10.1111/j.1526-4637.2010.01035.x

Minor, J. S., & Epstein, J. B. (2011a). Burning mouth syndrome and secondary oral burning. *Otolaryngologic Clinics of North America.* http://doi.org/10.1016/j.otc.2010.09.008

Minor, J. S., & Epstein, J. B. (2011b). Burning mouth syndrome and secondary oral burning. *Otolaryngol Clin N Am, 44*(1), 205–19, vii. http://doi.org/10.1016/j.otc.2010.09.008

Mock, D., & Chugh, D. (2010). Burning mouth syndrome. *Int.J.Oral Sci., 2*(1), 1–4.

Mock, D., & Chugh, D. (2010). Burning mouth syndrome. *International Journal of Oral Science, 2*(1), 1–4. http://doi.org/10.4248/IJOS10008

Muzyka, B. C., & De Rossi, S. S. (1999). A review of burning mouth syndrome. *Cutis; Cutaneous Medicine for the Practitioner, 64*(1), 29–35.

Ni Riordain, R., Moloney, E., Osullivan, K., & McCreary, C. (2010). Burning mouth syndrome and oral health-related quality of life: Is there a change over time? *Oral Diseases, 16*(7), 643–647. http://doi.org/10.1111/j.1601-0825.2010.01666.x

Patton, L. L., Siegel, M. A., Benoliel, R., & De Laat, A. (2007). Management of burning mouth syndrome: systematic review and management recommendations. *Oral Surgery, Oral Medicine, Oral Pathology, Oral Radiology, and Endodontics, 103 Suppl*, S39.e1–e13. http://doi.org/10.1016/j.tripleo.2006.11.009

Rhodus, N. L., Carlson, C. R., & Miller, C. S. (2003). Burning mouth (syndrome) disorder. *Quintessence International (Berlin, Germany : 1985), 34*(8), 587–593.

Salort Llorca, C., Mínguez Serra, M. P., & Silvestre, F. J. (2008). Drug-induced burning mouth syndrome: A new etiological diagnosis. *Medicina*

Oral, Patologia Oral Y Cirugia Bucal, 13(3), 167–170.
http://doi.org/10488787 [pii]

Savage, N. W., Boras, V. V, & Barker, K. (2006). Burning mouth syndrome:
clinical presentation, diagnosis and treatment. *The Australasian Journal of
Dermatology, 47*(2), 77–81; quiz 82–83. http://doi.org/10.1111/j.1440-
0960.2006.00236.x

Spanemberg, J. C., Cherubini, K., De Figueiredo, M. A. Z., Yurgel, L. S., &
Salum, F. G. (2012). Aetiology and therapeutics of burning mouth syndrome:
An update. *Gerodontology.* http://doi.org/10.1111/j.1741-2358.2010.00384.x

Speciali, J. G., & Stuginski-Barbosa, J. (2008). Burning mouth syndrome.
Current Pain and Headache Reports. http://doi.org/10.1007/s11916-008-
0047-9

Stuginski-Barbosa, J., Rodrigues, G. G. R., Bigal, M. E., & Speciali, J. G.
(2008). Burning mouth syndrome responsive to pramipexol. *Journal of
Headache and Pain, 9*(1), 43–45. http://doi.org/10.1007/s10194-008-0003-4

Suda, S., Takagai, S., Inoshima-Takahashi, K., Sugihara, G., Mori, N., &
Takei, N. (2008). Electroconvulsive therapy for burning mouth syndrome.
Acta Psychiatrica Scandinavica, 118(6), 503–504.
http://doi.org/10.1111/j.1600-0447.2008.01261.x

Sun, A., Wu, K.-M., Wang, Y.-P., Lin, H.-P., Chen, H.-M., & Chiang, C.-P.
(2013). Burning mouth syndrome: a review and update. *Journal of Oral
Pathology & Medicine : Official Publication of the International Association
of Oral Pathologists and the American Academy of Oral Pathology, 42*, 649–
55. http://doi.org/10.1111/jop.12101

Thoppay, J. R., De Rossi, S. S., & Ciarrocca, K. N. (2013). Burning mouth
syndrome. *Dental Clinics of North America.*
http://doi.org/10.1016/j.cden.2013.04.010

Torgerson, R. R. (2010). Burning mouth syndrome. *Dermatologic Therapy.*
http://doi.org/10.1111/j.1529-8019.2010.01325.x

Wandeur, T., De Moura, S. A. B., De Medeiros, A. M. C., MacHado, M. A.
N., De Azevedo Alanis, L. R., Grégio, A. M. T., … De Lima, A. A. S.
(2011). Exfoliative cytology of the oral mucosa in burning mouth syndrome:
A cytomorphological and cytomorphometric analysis. *Gerodontology, 28*(1),
44–48. http://doi.org/10.1111/j.1741-2358.2009.00319.x

Zur, E. (2012). Burning mouth syndrome: a discussion of a complex pathology. *International Journal of Pharmaceutical Compounding, 16*(3), 196–205. Retrieved from http://www.ncbi.nlm.nih.gov/pubmed/23050296\nhttp://www.scopus.com/inw eid=2-s2.0-84868250574&partnerID=tZOtx3y1

Burning Mouth Syndrome Internet Articles and Research

Burning Mouth Syndrome (Glossopyrosis) Medication | Drugs.com. (2015). Retrieved on January 22, 2015, from http://www.drugs.com/condition/burning-mouth-syndrome.html.

Burning Mouth Syndrome: Learn About Symptoms. (2015). Retrieved on January 22, 2015, from http://www.medicinenet.com/burning_mouth_syndrome/article.htm.

Burning Mouth Syndrome. (2015). Retrieved on January 22, 2015, from http://emedicine.medscape.com/article/1508869-overview.

Burning Mouth Syndrome. (2015). Retrieved on January 22, 2015, from http://www.aafp.org/afp/2002/0215/p615.html.

Burning Mouth Syndrome. (2015). Retrieved on January 22, 2015, from http://www.nidcr.nih.gov/oralhealth/Topics/Burning/BurningMouthSyndrome

Burning Tongue Syndrome | 34. (2015). Retrieved on January 22, 2015, from http://www.34-menopause-symptoms.com/burning-tongue/articles/burning-tongue-syndrome.htm.

Burning mouth syndrome (stomatodynia) | QJM: An International …. (2015). Retrieved on January 22, 2015, from http://qjmed.oxfordjournals.org/content/100/8/527.

Burning mouth syndrome. (2015). Retrieved on January 22, 2015, from http://en.wikipedia.org/wiki/Burning_mouth_syndrome.

Laser acupuncture in the treatment of burning mouth syndrome: a …. (2015). Retrieved on January 22, 2015, from http://aim.bmj.com/content/31/4/453.short?rss=1.

MayoClinic.com Health Library. (2015). Retrieved on January 22, 2015, from http://www.riversideonline.com/health_reference/dental-care/ds00462.cfm.

Oral burning symptoms and burning mouth syndrome. (2015). Retrieved on January 22, 2015, from http://scielo.isciii.es/scielo.php?pid=S1698-

69462006000300007&script=sci_arttext.

burning mouth syndrome. (2015). Retrieved on January 22, 2015, from http://medical-dictionary.thefreedictionary.com/burning+mouth+syndrome.

Scott Moses, MD. (2015). *Burning Mouth Syndrome.* Retrieved on January 22, 2015, from http://www.fpnotebook.com/ent/sx/BrngMthSyndrm.htm.

Suarez P and Clark GT. (2015). *Burning mouth syndrome: an update on diagnosis and treatment ....* Retrieved on January 22, 2015, from http://www.ncbi.nlm.nih.gov/pubmed/16967671.

CHAPTER 3

EPIDEMIOLOGY

Epidemiology is the branch of medicine concerned with researching factors related to the distribution of disease in human populations. Important components of epidemiological research include studying the cause, incidence, prevalence, behavior, and transmission of disease affecting groups of people. Epidemiology is most often associated with public health since it is primarily concerned with disease outbreaks in human populations, in contrast to disease manifestation in individuals. Depending on research needs, the population studied can be of any size and composition as long members of the group share specific characteristics important to the researcher. For instance, study populations can be based on geography, where populations as large as individual nations or entire continents are examined. Conversely, populations may be as small a remote village or a single work site where all individuals are exposed to identical environmental toxins, such as airborne coal dust inhaled by workers at a local coal mine. While geography is often an important consideration in epidemiological research, groups can also be studied based on numerous factors unrelated to physical location, such as age, gender, race or nationality, diet, and so on.

Since epidemiology and pathology both study disease, people often find it difficult to distinguish between the two scientific disciplines. One easy, albeit vastly oversimplified way to distinguish between the two disciplines, is that epidemiology is the study of disease in groups of people while pathology studies disease in an individual person or organism.

Morbidity and Disease

Two of the most basic and important concepts in Epidemiology are incidence and prevalence. Incidence and prevalence are both measures of morbidity. Quite simply, morbidity is **the extent of illness, injury or disability in a defined population**. In epidemiology, incidence and prevalence are important in that both statistics attempt to measure risk, where risk is **the likelihood that an individual within a population will contract a disease**. While both incidence and prevalence attempt to estimate the occurrence of a health condition during a specified period of time, many people confuse incidence and prevalence and use them interchangeably falsely assuming that one is simply a synonym for the other. However, when researching Burning Mouth Syndrome it is important to remember that each term has its own distinct meaning.

The term incidence refers to the number of new cases of a health condition in a given time period. In other words, incidence most closely resembles the number of new diagnoses. Conversely, prevalence means the number of persons *currently* suffering from a health condition. In this regard, a person diagnosed with a *chronic* health condition (where *chronic* describes an illness persisting over a long time period) will be included in incidence statistics in only one year, that being the year they were diagnosed but this same individual will be included prevalence reports each year they suffer this health condition. Taken one step further, a newly diagnosed patient will be counted in both incidence and prevalence statistics during the patient's first year of a health condition but in subsequent years will only be included in prevalence statistics. The important takeaway, therefore, is that for any given timeframe the prevalance of a health condition will always be equal or greater than the incidence of the same condition. Most of the time incidence and prevalence statistics are reported on an annual basis, though for health conditions like Influenza seasonal or monthly morbidity may be more important.

Because these two concepts have distinct meanings they are most revealing taken together and often the two numbers can vary dramatically from one another. For short-lived health conditions like Influenza incidence can be very high during years with large outbreaks as large populations may suffer from a vaccine resistant Influenza strain but the overall prevalence may be quite low in subsequent years. On the other hand, for some chronic illnesses the incidence rate may be low when compared to the prevalence rate. An example is when public health researchers introduce new preventative treatment strategies for a certain health condition. Currently, enormous resources are being used to prevent Type II Diabetes. Why? Because in recent years there has been a dramatic rise in the number of individuals diagnosed with this disease, resulting in a large number of individuals managing Diabetes in any given year. However, if preventative efforts are successful we can expect the number of new diagnoses in the first "successful" year to decline dramatically. Therefore, in that year the incidence of the disease will significantly decline but those already afflicted with the disease may still keep the prevalence statistics high.

Thus, when reviewing incidence and prevalence statistics it is worthwhile to compare the figures over more than one year. If, for example, you notice that incidence and prevalence rates are both high for nine (9) consecutive years but the incidence rate drops dramatically in the tenth year you may rightly hypothesize that a new preventative treatment was introduced in the tenth year therefore leading you to research your assumption further.

It is also important to remember that incidence and prevalence statistics do not attempt to measure the entire population. Instead these statistics generally only measure populations at risk. To illustrate, incidence and prevalence measures of Cervical Cancer only include women. Likewise, Testicular Cancer is only calculated for men. While this is important to remember, the research you will discover will clearly report the population the estimate is intended to reflect.

Mathematically, with "/" meaning "divided by" the calculations for incidence and prevalence can be expressed as follows:

Incidence Rate = Number of New Cases within a Given Time Period / Number of People at Risk of Getting the Disease

Prevalence Rate = Total Number of Cases at a Single Point in Time / Number of People at Risk of Getting the Disease

Multiply the the result by 100 or 1000 to get the number of person to get the number of cases per 100 or 1000, respectively.

Finally, remember that incidence and prevalence statistics are only estimates and a not a perfectly exact reflection of the population being measured. For example, for some health disorders the the incidence rate can be greater than the actual number of people affected by a health condition. A typical example is incidence reports for the common cold. Many individuals may get a common cold two or more times in a given year and therefore will be counted multiple times in incidence statistics even though they are only one person. Likewise, some prevalence measures estimating the occurrence of a particular cancer type, for instance, may include persons in remission where other prevalence estimates do not. Thus, when reviewing incidence and prevalence reports it is important to not only understand the limitations of each but also the methodology researchers used to report a final estimate.

Sources of Morbidity Statistics

Morbidity statistics are aggregated and collected by a number of organizations. Some organizations that collect this data include:

1. Hospitals and clinics
2. Disease and cancer registries
3. Communicable disease reporting surveillance public health agencies
4. Vital statistics
5. Surveys
6. Health and life insurance plans

Mortality and Disease

One final important indicator of the health status of populations is mortality. Mortality literally means "death" and therefore a mortality rate is the percentage of death in a population in any given time. Importantly, there are a number of mortality rates including, but not limited to, the child mortality rate, infant mortality rate, maternal mortality rate, and age-specific mortality. The crude mortality rate is simply the total number of deaths per 1,000 people, regardless of age, gender, disease, etc. Therefore, the calculation of the crude mortality rate is:

Annual Mortality Rate from All Causes = (Total Number of Deaths in One Year from All Causes / Number of Persons in Population at Mid-Year) x 1,000

Where "/" means "divided by" and "*" means "multiplied by" and the part of formula enclosed in parentheses "( )" is to be performed first.

Sources of Mortality Statistics

The Centers for Disease Control and Prevention (CDC) is the agency that oversees public health in the United States. While the National Institutes of Health is the nation's primary health care research agency, the CDC primary focus is on the health of the population as a whole, and instead of researching disease concentrates instead on the prevention and control of disease outbreaks by primarily studying disease transmission. CDC online resources provide basic information about illness and disease but focus on communicating information about the impact of health conditions on large populations. A vast amount of text and data are available on the CDC website at http://www.cdc.gov/

Most mortality statistics are derived from data from individual death certificates. Primary on death certificates is the identification of the cause of death, frequently abbreviated as COD. Death certificates in the United States generally report two CODs, an **immediate COD** and an **underlying COD**. For example, for leukemia patients a common immediate cause of death is sepsis caused by the underlying cause of death, leukemia.

In the United States, aggregated mortality data and statistics can be found by searching:

1. The **National Death Index (NDI)** from the National Center for Health Statistics http://www.cdc.gov/nchs/ndi.htm

2. The **Morbidity and Mortality Weekly Report** from the Centers for Disease Control and Prevention (CDC) http://www.cdc.gov/mmwr/

3. State vital records. Links to each state agency responsible for that state's vital records can be found at http://www.cdc.gov/nchs/w2w.htm

4. Tumor registries. Links to tumor registries can be found at http://apps.nccd.cdc.gov/dcpc_Programs

Burning Mouth Syndrome Journal Articles

Al Quran, F. A. M. (2004). Psychological profile in burning mouth syndrome. *Oral Surgery, Oral Medicine, Oral Pathology, Oral Radiology, and Endodontics, 97*(3), 339–344. http://doi.org/10.1016/j.tripleo.2003.09.017

Baharvand, M., & Hemmati, F. (2006). Frequency of subjective dry mouth and burning mouth syndrome in elder residents of sanitariums in Tehran, 2005 [Farsi]. *Journal of Islamic Dental Association of Iran, 18*, 13.

Balasubramaniam, R., Klasser, G. D., & Delcanho, R. (2009). Separating oral burning from burning mouth syndrome: Unravelling a diagnostic enigma. *Australian Dental Journal.* http://doi.org/10.1111/j.1834-7819.2009.01153.x

Barker, K. E., & Savage, N. W. (2005). Burning mouth syndrome: An update on recent findings. *Australian Dental Journal.* http://doi.org/10.1111/j.1834-7819.2005.tb00363.x

Boy-Metin, Z., Kayhan, K. B., & Unur, M. (2008). Burning mouth syndrome. *Kulak Burun Bogaz Ihtis Derg, 18*(3), 188–196. Retrieved from http://www.ncbi.nlm.nih.gov/pubmed/18985004

Boy-Metin, Z., Kayhan, K. B., & Unür, M. (2008). Burning mouth syndrome. *Kulak Burun Boğaz Ihtisas Dergisi : KBB = Journal of Ear, Nose, and Throat, 18*(3), 188–96. Retrieved from http://www.ncbi.nlm.nih.gov/pubmed/19388467

Brufau-Redondo, C., Martín-Brufau, R., Corbalán-Velez, R., & De Concepción-Salesa, a. (2002). Burning mouth syndrome. *British Dental Journal, 45*(6), 237–241. http://doi.org/10.1111/j.1526-4637.2010.01035.x

Cerchiari, D. P., de Moricz, R. D., Sanjar, F. A., Rapoport, P. B., Moretti, G., & Guerra, M. M. (2006). Burning mouth syndrome: etiology. *Brazilian Journal of Otorhinolaryngology, 72*(3), 419–23. http://doi.org/S0034-72992006000300021 [pii]

Cibirka, R. M., Nelson, S. K., & Lefebvre, C. A. (1999). A review of burning mouth syndrome. *The Journal of Prosthetic Dentistry, 78*(1), 29–35.

Coon, E. A., & Laughlin, R. S. (2012). Burning mouth syndrome in Parkinson's disease: Dopamine as cure or cause? *Journal of Headache and Pain, 13*(3), 255–257. http://doi.org/10.1007/s10194-012-0421-1

Crow, H. C., & Gonzalez, Y. (2012). Burning Mouth Syndrome. *Oral and*

Maxillofacial Surgery Clinics of North America, 65(5), 343–347.
http://doi.org/10.4248/IJOS10008

Crow, H. C., & Gonzalez, Y. (2013). Burning Mouth Syndrome. *Oral and Maxillofacial Surgery Clinics of North America.*
http://doi.org/10.1016/j.coms.2012.11.001

Fedele, S., Fricchione, G., Porter, & Mignogna, M. (2007a). Stomatodynia or burning mouth syndrome. *Acta Dermatovenerologica Croatica ADC Hrvatsko Dermatolosko Drustvo*, 100(4), 231–235. Retrieved from http://discovery.ucl.ac.uk/148057/

Fedele, S., Fricchione, G., Porter, S. R., & Mignogna, M. D. (2007b). Stomatodynia or burning mouth syndrome. *Acta Dermatovenerologica Croatica ADC Hrvatsko Dermatolosko Drustvo*, 11(4), 231–235. Retrieved from http://discovery.ucl.ac.uk/148057/

Friedman, D. I. (2010). Topirimate-induced burning mouth syndrome. *Headache*, 50(8), 1383–1385. http://doi.org/10.1111/j.1526-4610.2010.01720.x

Gerlinger, I. (2012). [Burning sensation in oral cavity--burning mouth syndrome in everyday medical practice]. *Ideggyógyászati Szemle*, 65(9-10), 295–301. Retrieved from http://www.ncbi.nlm.nih.gov/pubmed/23126213

Grushka, M., Epstein, J. B., & Gorsky, M. (2002). Burning mouth syndrome. *American Family Physician*, 65(4). http://doi.org/10.3748/wjg.v19.i5.665

Grushka, M., Epstein, J. B., & Gorsky, M. (2002). Burning mouth syndrome. *Am Fam Physician*, 65(4), 615–620. Retrieved from http://www.ncbi.nlm.nih.gov/entrez/query.fcgi?
cmd=Retrieve&db=PubMed&dopt=Citation&list_uids=11871678

Gurvits, G. E., & Tan, A. (2013). Burning mouth syndrome. *World Journal of Gastroenterology : WJG*, 19(5), 665–72.
http://doi.org/10.3748/wjg.v19.i5.665

Hagelberg, N., Forssell, H., Rinne, J. O., Scheinin, H., Taiminen, T., Aalto, S., … Jääskeläinen, S. (2003). Striatal dopamine D1 and D2 receptors in burning mouth syndrome. *Pain*, 101(1-2), 149–154.
http://doi.org/10.1016/S0304-3959(02)00323-8

Hens, M. J., Alonso-Ferreira, V., Villaverde-Hueso, A., Abaitua, I., & Posada De La Paz, M. (2012). Cost-effectiveness analysis of burning mouth syndrome therapy. *Community Dentistry and Oral Epidemiology, 40*(2), 185–192. http://doi.org/10.1111/j.1600-0528.2011.00645.x

Huang, W., Rothe, M. J., & Grant-Kels, J. M. (1996). The burning mouth syndrome. *Journal of the American Academy of Dermatology, 34*(1), 91–98. http://doi.org/10.1016/S0190-9622(96)90840-3

Jääskeläinen, S. K. (2012). Pathophysiology of primary burning mouth syndrome. *Clinical Neurophysiology.* http://doi.org/10.1016/j.clinph.2011.07.054

Klasser, G. D., Epstein, J. B., & Villines, D. (2011). Management of burning mouth syndrome. *Journal (Canadian Dental Association), 77*, b151. Retrieved from http://www.ncbi.nlm.nih.gov/pubmed/22260804

Klasser, G. D., Fischer, D. J., & Epstein, J. B. (2008). Burning Mouth Syndrome: Recognition, Understanding, and Management. *Oral and Maxillofacial Surgery Clinics of North America.* http://doi.org/10.1016/j.coms.2007.12.012

Lamey, P. J., & Lamb, A. B. (1994). Lip component of burning mouth syndrome. *Oral Surgery, Oral Medicine, and Oral Pathology, 78*(5), 590–593. http://doi.org/10.1016/0030-4220(94)90169-4

Lauria, G., Majorana, A., Borgna, M., Lombardi, R., Penza, P., Padovani, A., & Sapelli, P. (2005). Trigeminal small-fiber sensory neuropathy causes burning mouth syndrome. *Pain, 115*(3), 332–337. http://doi.org/10.1016/j.pain.2005.03.028

López-Jornet, P., Camacho-Alonso, F., & Andujar-Mateos, P. (2011). A prospective, randomized study on the efficacy of tongue protector in patients with burning mouth syndrome. *Oral Diseases, 17*(3), 277–282. http://doi.org/10.1111/j.1601-0825.2010.01737.x

López-Jornet, P., Camacho-Alonso, F., Andujar-Mateos, P., Sánchez-Siles, M., & Gómez-Garcia, F. (2010). Burning mouth syndrome: an update. *Medicina Oral, Patología Oral Y Cirugía Bucal, 15*(4), e562–8. Retrieved from http://www.ncbi.nlm.nih.gov/pubmed/23772971

Marino, R., Capaccio, P., Pignataro, L., & Spadari, F. (2009). Burning mouth syndrome: The role of contact hypersensitivity. *Oral Diseases, 15*(4), 255–258. http://doi.org/10.1111/j.1601-0825.2009.01515.x

Marino, R., Torretta, S., Capaccio, P., Pignataro, L., & Spadari, F. (2010).

Different therapeutic strategies for burning mouth syndrome: preliminary data. *Journal of Oral Pathology & Medicine : Official Publication of the International Association of Oral Pathologists and the American Academy of Oral Pathology, 39*(8), 611–616. http://doi.org/10.1111/j.1600-0714.2010.00922.x

Mignogna, M. D., Adamo, D., Schiavone, V., Ravel, M. G., & Fortuna, G. (2011). Burning Mouth Syndrome Responsive to Duloxetine: A Case Report. *Pain Medicine, 12*(3), 466–469. http://doi.org/10.1111/j.1526-4637.2010.01035.x

Minor, J. S., & Epstein, J. B. (2011a). Burning mouth syndrome and secondary oral burning. *Otolaryngologic Clinics of North America.* http://doi.org/10.1016/j.otc.2010.09.008

Minor, J. S., & Epstein, J. B. (2011b). Burning mouth syndrome and secondary oral burning. *Otolaryngol Clin N Am, 44*(1), 205–19, vii. http://doi.org/10.1016/j.otc.2010.09.008

Mock, D., & Chugh, D. (2010). Burning mouth syndrome. *Int.J.Oral Sci., 2*(1), 1–4.

Mock, D., & Chugh, D. (2010). Burning mouth syndrome. *International Journal of Oral Science, 2*(1), 1–4. http://doi.org/10.4248/IJOS10008

Muzyka, B. C., & De Rossi, S. S. (1999). A review of burning mouth syndrome. *Cutis; Cutaneous Medicine for the Practitioner, 64*(1), 29–35.

Ni Riordain, R., Moloney, E., Osullivan, K., & McCreary, C. (2010). Burning mouth syndrome and oral health-related quality of life: Is there a change over time? *Oral Diseases, 16*(7), 643–647. http://doi.org/10.1111/j.1601-0825.2010.01666.x

Patton, L. L., Siegel, M. A., Benoliel, R., & De Laat, A. (2007). Management of burning mouth syndrome: systematic review and management recommendations. *Oral Surgery, Oral Medicine, Oral Pathology, Oral Radiology, and Endodontics, 103 Suppl*, S39.e1–e13. http://doi.org/10.1016/j.tripleo.2006.11.009

Savage, N. W., Boras, V. V, & Barker, K. (2006). Burning mouth syndrome: clinical presentation, diagnosis and treatment. *The Australasian Journal of Dermatology, 47*(2), 77–81; quiz 82–83. http://doi.org/10.1111/j.1440-0960.2006.00236.x

Spanemberg, J. C., Cherubini, K., De Figueiredo, M. A. Z., Yurgel, L. S., & Salum, F. G. (2012). Aetiology and therapeutics of burning mouth syndrome: An update. *Gerodontology*. http://doi.org/10.1111/j.1741-2358.2010.00384.x

Speciali, J. G., & Stuginski-Barbosa, J. (2008). Burning mouth syndrome. *Current Pain and Headache Reports*. http://doi.org/10.1007/s11916-008-0047-9

Speciali, J. G., & Stuginski-Barbosa, J. (2008). Burning mouth syndrome. *Curr Pain Headache Rep.*, *12*(4), 279–284.

Stuginski-Barbosa, J., Rodrigues, G. G. R., Bigal, M. E., & Speciali, J. G. (2008). Burning mouth syndrome responsive to pramipexol. *Journal of Headache and Pain*, *9*(1), 43–45. http://doi.org/10.1007/s10194-008-0003-4

Sun, A., Wu, K.-M., Wang, Y.-P., Lin, H.-P., Chen, H.-M., & Chiang, C.-P. (2013). Burning mouth syndrome: a review and update. *Journal of Oral Pathology & Medicine : Official Publication of the International Association of Oral Pathologists and the American Academy of Oral Pathology*, *42*, 649–55. http://doi.org/10.1111/jop.12101

Thoppay, J. R., De Rossi, S. S., & Ciarrocca, K. N. (2013). Burning mouth syndrome. *Dental Clinics of North America*. http://doi.org/10.1016/j.cden.2013.04.010

Torgerson, R. R. (2010). Burning mouth syndrome. *Dermatologic Therapy*. http://doi.org/10.1111/j.1529-8019.2010.01325.x

Wandeur, T., De Moura, S. A. B., De Medeiros, A. M. C., MacHado, M. A. N., De Azevedo Alanis, L. R., Grégio, A. M. T., … De Lima, A. A. S. (2011). Exfoliative cytology of the oral mucosa in burning mouth syndrome: A cytomorphological and cytomorphometric analysis. *Gerodontology*, *28*(1), 44–48. http://doi.org/10.1111/j.1741-2358.2009.00319.x

Witt, E., & Palla, S. (2002). Mundbrennen, [Burning mouth]. *Schmerz (Berlin, Germany)*, *16*(5), 389–94. http://doi.org/10.1007/s00482-002-0149-y

Zur, E. (2012). Burning mouth syndrome: a discussion of a complex pathology. *International Journal of Pharmaceutical Compounding*, *16*(3), 196–205. Retrieved from http://www.ncbi.nlm.nih.gov/pubmed/23050296\nhttp://www.scopus.com/inw eid=2-s2.0-84868250574&partnerID=tZOtx3y1

Burning Mouth Syndrome Internet Articles and Research

Bruxism: Signs And Symptoms. (2015). Retrieved on January 22, 2015, from http://www.colgateprofessional.com/patient-education/articles/bruxism-signs-and-symptoms.

Burning Mouth Syndrome and Menopause. (2015). Retrieved on January 22, 2015, from http://www.ncbi.nlm.nih.gov/pmc/articles/PMC3570906/.

Burning Mouth Syndrome. (2015). Retrieved on January 22, 2015, from http://www.nidcr.nih.gov/oralhealth/Topics/Burning/BurningMouthSyndrome

Burning Mouth Syndrome. (2015). Retrieved on January 22, 2015, from http://www.practicalpainmanagement.com/pain/maxillofacial/burning-mouth-syndrome.

Burning mouth syndrome, Type 1 Symptoms, Diagnosis, Treatments .... (2015). Retrieved on January 22, 2015, from http://www.rightdiagnosis.com/b/burning_mouth_syndrome_type_1/intro.htm

Burning mouth syndrome, Type 2 Symptoms, Diagnosis, Treatments .... (2015). Retrieved on January 22, 2015, from http://www.rightdiagnosis.com/b/burning_mouth_syndrome_type_2/intro.htm

Burning mouth syndrome. DermNet NZ. (2015). Retrieved on January 22, 2015, from http://www.dermnetnz.org/site-age-specific/burning-mouth.html.

Burning mouth syndrome: clinical profile of Brazilian patients. (2015). Retrieved on January 22, 2015, from http://www.scielo.br/scielo.php?script=sci_arttext&pid=S0103-64402007000400013.

Burning mouth syndrome: etiology. (2015). Retrieved on January 22, 2015, from http://www.scielo.br/scielo.php?pid=s0034-72992006000300021&script=sci_arttext&tlng=en.

Burning mouth syndrome. (2015). Retrieved on January 22, 2015, from http://en.wikipedia.org/wiki/Burning_mouth_syndrome.

Burning mouth syndrome. (2015). Retrieved on January 22, 2015, from http://www.rightdiagnosis.com/b/burning_mouth_syndrome_type_3/intro.htm

Home Remedies for Burning Tongue: Causes, Treatment .... (2015). Retrieved on January 22, 2015, from http://www.home-remedies-for-you.com/remedy/Burning-Tongue.html.

Managing a patient with burning mouth syndrome. (2015). Retrieved on January 22, 2015, from http://fg.bmj.com/content/early/2014/06/17/flgastro-2014-100431.abstract.

The Prevalence of Burning Mouth Syndrome: A Population. (2015). Retrieved on January 22, 2015, from http://onlinelibrary.wiley.com/doi/10.1111/bjd.13613/abstract.

Aegis Communications, By Gary D. Klasser, DMD. (2015). *Inside Dentistry – Burning Mouth Syndrome Linked to Menopause.* Retrieved on January 22, 2015, from http://www.dentalaegis.com/id/2011/10/burning-mouth-syndrome-linked-to-menopause.

Life Enhancement Products. (2015). *Lipoic Acid Helps Quench the Fire of Burning Mouth Syndrome.* Retrieved on January 22, 2015, from http://www.life-enhancement.com/magazine/article/726-lipoic-acid-helps-quench-the-fire-of-burning-mouth-syndrome.

Mignogna MD , et al.. (2015). *Unexplained somatic comorbidities in patients with burning mouth ....* Retrieved on January 22, 2015, from http://www.ncbi.nlm.nih.gov/pubmed/21528120.

wpadmin. (2015). *Home Remedies for Burning Mouth Syndrome | HRF.* Retrieved on January 22, 2015, from http://healthresearchfunding.org/home-remedies-burning-mouth-syndrome/.

CHAPTER 4

RISK FACTORS

&

CAUSES

During the course of researching health conditions many people use the the concepts of risk factors and causes interchangeably. However, it is important to remember in medicine these concepts have unique meanings. This Chapter will define these commonly confused concepts and explain the risk factors and causes of Burning Mouth Syndrome.

Risk Factors for Disease

A risk factor is any aspect or circumstance in a person's life that predisposes or makes it more likely that the person will acquire a particular health condition. Essentially, risk factors are anything that increases the chance of developing a disease. Some examples of risk factors for many diseases include age, a family history of certain conditions, use of tobacco products, being exposed to radiation or certain chemicals, infection with certain viruses or bacteria, and certain genetic makeups.

If you discover you have a risk factor for a certain condition it doesn't necessarily mean that you will get that disease. It only means your chances of the getting the disease are higher when compared to other individuals similar to yourself who are not exposed to the stated risk factor(s). In this regard, it is important to note that risk factors and causes are essentially measures of **correlation** or **causation**. The distinction between correlation and causation is very important in medical research.

Correlation means two factors are related and also expresses in statistical terms how closely the two factors are related. For example, there exists a correlation between age and food allergies, as children are about twice as likely as adults of having food allergies. However, this doesn't mean that being a child *causes* food allergies.

Causes of Disease

This leads us to the definition of causation and the dual nature of cause and effect. In medicine causation essentially implies change in the normal constitution or functioning of the body as the result of the introduction of a second factor (the cause). To return to the the previous example, food allergies are most commonly due to an allergen-antibody interaction, therefore the cause can be said to be the allergen-antibody interaction and the effect (or manifestation of the cause) is the food allergy (and not being a child). Researchers have discovered the reason that children are more likely to have food allergies is because their immune systems are not as well-developed as adults and their bodies are more likely to mistakenly identify certain foods as "harmful" and trigger the allergen-antibody reaction.

Similarly, when studying risk factors, another important terminology distinction is between **effect** and **association**. Both effect and association are quantitative measures of the increased or decreased prevalence, rate, or risk for disease in an exposed population but epidemiologists use the term effect when the risk factor can be changed and association when it cannot be changed. For example, one effect of obesity may be uterine cancer but this risk factor can be reduced or eliminated by losing weight. On the other hand, uterine cancer is only associated with women, but even though a hysterectomy will remove the uterus the patient will still remain a woman.

Most research you come across will clearly distinguish between correlation/causation and effect/association. Further, as you will soon discover, nearly all advances in research into illness and disease first establish correlation or association but only later establish causation or effect. For example, through observation researchers were able to quickly ascertain that smokers were more likely to develop lung cancer, meaning that there exists a correlation between smoking and lung cancer and was higher than between non-smoking and lung cancer. However, further research was needed to determine that smoking, and not some other attribute common among smokers, was a cause of lung cancer.

An extreme, and intuitively far-fetched but common example to illustrate our point is the story of Inept Researcher A. Among office workers, Inept Researcher A notices that workers who take many rest breaks have more sick days due to respiratory illness than workers who take fewer breaks. Inept Researcher A quickly concludes that "work breaks cause respiratory disease" and in his haste forgoes peer-reviewed journals and publishes his "landmark discovery" on his own, including a recommendation that government move quickly to establish laws prohibiting all work rest breaks. Soon, however,

All-Star Researcher B reads the article and does her own analysis of the data. In no time at all, All-Star Researcher B is able to debunk Inept Researcher A's conclusions by correctly determining that work breaks do not cause respiratory illness. She further hypothesizes (and is later proven correct) it is not the break itself causing respiratory illness; but what people do on these work breaks, namely smoking cigarettes that is the real cause of respiratory illness in persons taking frequent work breaks.

While Inept Researcher A's "discovery" may seem intuitively false, it is not always this easy to correctly identify incorrect or illogical conclusions of cause and effect. Therefore, during the course of your research take special note to distinguish statements of correlation with assertions of cause and effect or be prepared to suffer consequences of falsely jumping to erroneous conclusions.

Burning Mouth Syndrome Journal Articles

Abetz, L. M., & Savage, N. W. (2009). Burning mouth syndrome and psychological disorders. *Australian Dental Journal, 54*(2), 84–93; quiz 173. http://doi.org/10.1111/j.1834-7819.2009.01099.x

Afrin, L. B. Burning mouth syndrome and mast cell activation disorder., 111 Oral surgery, oral medicine, oral pathology, oral radiology, and endodontics 465–472 (2011). http://doi.org/10.1016/j.tripleo.2010.11.030

Balasubramaniam, R., Klasser, G. D., & Delcanho, R. (2009). Separating oral burning from burning mouth syndrome: Unravelling a diagnostic enigma. *Australian Dental Journal.* http://doi.org/10.1111/j.1834-7819.2009.01153.x

Barker, K. E., Batstone, M. D., & Savage, N. W. (2009). Comparison of treatment modalities in burning mouth syndrome. *Australian Dental Journal, 54*(4), 300–305. http://doi.org/10.1111/j.1834-7819.2009.01154.x

Barker, K. E., & Savage, N. W. (2005). Burning mouth syndrome: An update on recent findings. *Australian Dental Journal.* http://doi.org/10.1111/j.1834-7819.2005.tb00363.x

Boy-Metin, Z., Kayhan, K. B., & Unür, M. (2008). Burning mouth syndrome. *Kulak Burun Boğaz Ihtisas Dergisi : KBB = Journal of Ear, Nose, and Throat, 18*(3), 188–96. Retrieved from http://www.ncbi.nlm.nih.gov/pubmed/19388467

Brufau-Redondo, C., Martín-Brufau, R., Corbalán-Velez, R., & De Concepción-Salesa, a. (2002). Burning mouth syndrome. *British Dental Journal, 45*(6), 237–241. http://doi.org/10.1111/j.1526-4637.2010.01035.x

Brufau-Redondo, C., Martin-Brufau, R., Corbalan-Velez, R., & de Concepcion-Salesa, A. (2008). {[}Burning mouth syndrome{]}. *Actas Dermosifiliogr, 99*(6), 431–440.

Cerchiari, D. P., de Moricz, R. D., Sanjar, F. A., Rapoport, P. B., Moretti, G., & Guerra, M. M. (2006). Burning mouth syndrome: etiology. *Brazilian Journal of Otorhinolaryngology, 72*(3), 419–23. http://doi.org/S0034-72992006000300021 [pii]

Cho, G. S., Han, M. W., Lee, B., Roh, J. L., Choi, S. H., Cho, K. J., … Kim, S. Y. (2010). Zinc deficiency may be a cause of burning mouth syndrome as zinc replacement therapy has therapeutic effects. *Journal of Oral Pathology and Medicine, 39*(9), 722–727. http://doi.org/10.1111/j.1600-

0714.2010.00914.x

Cibirka, R. M., Nelson, S. K., & Lefebvre, C. A. (1999). A review of burning mouth syndrome. *The Journal of Prosthetic Dentistry, 78*(1), 29–35.

Coon, E. A., & Laughlin, R. S. (2012). Burning mouth syndrome in Parkinson's disease: Dopamine as cure or cause? *Journal of Headache and Pain, 13*(3), 255–257. http://doi.org/10.1007/s10194-012-0421-1

Crow, H. C., & Gonzalez, Y. (2012). Burning Mouth Syndrome. *Oral and Maxillofacial Surgery Clinics of North America, 65*(5), 343–347. http://doi.org/10.4248/IJOS10008

Crow, H. C., & Gonzalez, Y. (2013). Burning Mouth Syndrome. *Oral and Maxillofacial Surgery Clinics of North America.* http://doi.org/10.1016/j.coms.2012.11.001

Ducasse, D., Courtet, P., & Olie, E. (2013). Burning mouth syndrome: current clinical, physiopathologic, and therapeutic data. *Regional Anesthesia and Pain Medicine, 38*(5), 380–90. http://doi.org/10.1097/AAP.0b013e3182a1f0db

Fedele, S., Fricchione, G., Porter, & Mignogna, M. (2007a). Stomatodynia or burning mouth syndrome. *Acta Dermatovenerologica Croatica ADC Hrvatsko Dermatolosko Drustvo, 100*(4), 231–235. Retrieved from http://discovery.ucl.ac.uk/148057/

Fedele, S., Fricchione, G., Porter, S. R., & Mignogna, M. D. (2007b). Stomatodynia or burning mouth syndrome. *Acta Dermatovenerologica Croatica ADC Hrvatsko Dermatolosko Drustvo, 11*(4), 231–235. Retrieved from http://discovery.ucl.ac.uk/148057/

Friedman, D. I. (2010). Topirimate-induced burning mouth syndrome. *Headache, 50*(8), 1383–1385. http://doi.org/10.1111/j.1526-4610.2010.01720.x

Grushka, M., Epstein, J. B., & Gorsky, M. (2002a). Burning mouth syndrome. *American Family Physician, 65*(4). http://doi.org/10.3748/wjg.v19.i5.665

Grushka, M., Epstein, J. B., & Gorsky, M. (2002). Burning mouth syndrome. *Am Fam Physician, 65*(4), 615–620. Retrieved from http://www.ncbi.nlm.nih.gov/entrez/query.fcgi?cmd=Retrieve&db=PubMed&dopt=Citation&list_uids=11871678

Grushka, M., Epstein, J. B., & Gorsky, M. (2003). Burning mouth syndrome and other oral sensory disorders: A unifying hypothesis. *Pain Research and Management.*

Grushka, M., Epstein, J., & Gorsky, M. (2002b). Burning mouth syndrome. *American Family Physician, 65*(4), 615–620. Retrieved from http://www.ncbi.nlm.nih.gov/pubmed/11871678

Gurvits, G. E., & Tan, A. (2013). Burning mouth syndrome. *World Journal of Gastroenterology : WJG, 19*(5), 665–72. http://doi.org/10.3748/wjg.v19.i5.665

Hagelberg, N., Forssell, H., Rinne, J. O., Scheinin, H., Taiminen, T., Aalto, S., … Jääskeläinen, S. (2003). Striatal dopamine D1 and D2 receptors in burning mouth syndrome. *Pain, 101*(1-2), 149–154. http://doi.org/10.1016/S0304-3959(02)00323-8

Huang, W., Rothe, M. J., & Grant-Kels, J. M. (1996). The burning mouth syndrome. *Journal of the American Academy of Dermatology, 34*(1), 91–98. http://doi.org/10.1016/S0190-9622(96)90840-3

Jääskeläinen, S. K. (2012). Pathophysiology of primary burning mouth syndrome. *Clinical Neurophysiology.* http://doi.org/10.1016/j.clinph.2011.07.054

Klasser, G. D., Epstein, J. B., & Villines, D. (2011). Management of burning mouth syndrome. *Journal (Canadian Dental Association), 77,* b151. Retrieved from http://www.ncbi.nlm.nih.gov/pubmed/22260804

Klasser, G. D., Fischer, D. J., & Epstein, J. B. (2008). Burning Mouth Syndrome: Recognition, Understanding, and Management. *Oral and Maxillofacial Surgery Clinics of North America.* http://doi.org/10.1016/j.coms.2007.12.012

Lamey, P. J., & Lamb, A. B. (1994). Lip component of burning mouth syndrome. *Oral Surgery, Oral Medicine, and Oral Pathology, 78*(5), 590–593. http://doi.org/10.1016/0030-4220(94)90169-4

Lauria, G., Majorana, A., Borgna, M., Lombardi, R., Penza, P., Padovani, A., & Sapelli, P. (2005). Trigeminal small-fiber sensory neuropathy causes burning mouth syndrome. *Pain, 115*(3), 332–337. http://doi.org/10.1016/j.pain.2005.03.028

López-Jornet, P., Camacho-Alonso, F., & Andujar-Mateos, P. (2011). A prospective, randomized study on the efficacy of tongue protector in patients with burning mouth syndrome. *Oral Diseases, 17*(3), 277–282. http://doi.org/10.1111/j.1601-0825.2010.01737.x

López-Jornet, P., Camacho-Alonso, F., Andujar-Mateos, P., Sánchez-Siles, M., & Gómez-Garcia, F. (2010). Burning mouth syndrome: an update. *Medicina Oral, Patología Oral Y Cirugía Bucal, 15*(4), e562–8. Retrieved from http://www.ncbi.nlm.nih.gov/pubmed/23772971

Marino, R., Capaccio, P., Pignataro, L., & Spadari, F. (2009). Burning mouth syndrome: The role of contact hypersensitivity. *Oral Diseases, 15*(4), 255–258. http://doi.org/10.1111/j.1601-0825.2009.01515.x

Marino, R., Torretta, S., Capaccio, P., Pignataro, L., & Spadari, F. (2010). Different therapeutic strategies for burning mouth syndrome: preliminary data. *Journal of Oral Pathology & Medicine : Official Publication of the International Association of Oral Pathologists and the American Academy of Oral Pathology, 39*(8), 611–616. http://doi.org/10.1111/j.1600-0714.2010.00922.x

Mignogna, M. D., Adamo, D., Schiavone, V., Ravel, M. G., & Fortuna, G. (2011). Burning Mouth Syndrome Responsive to Duloxetine: A Case Report. *Pain Medicine, 12*(3), 466–469. http://doi.org/10.1111/j.1526-4637.2010.01035.x

Minguez-Sanz, M.-P., Salort-Llorca, C., & Silvestre-Donat, F.-J. (2011). Etiology of burning mouth syndrome: a review and update. *Medicina Oral, Patología Oral Y Cirugía Bucal, 16*(2), e144–8. Retrieved from http://www.ncbi.nlm.nih.gov/pubmed/21217613

Minor, J. S., & Epstein, J. B. (2011a). Burning mouth syndrome and secondary oral burning. *Otolaryngologic Clinics of North America.* http://doi.org/10.1016/j.otc.2010.09.008

Minor, J. S., & Epstein, J. B. (2011b). Burning mouth syndrome and secondary oral burning. *Otolaryngol Clin N Am, 44*(1), 205–19, vii. http://doi.org/10.1016/j.otc.2010.09.008

Mock, D., & Chugh, D. (2010). Burning mouth syndrome. *International Journal of Oral Science, 2*(1), 1–4. http://doi.org/10.4248/IJOS10008

Muzyka, B. C., & De Rossi, S. S. (1999). A review of burning mouth syndrome. *Cutis; Cutaneous Medicine for the Practitioner, 64*(1), 29–35.

Ni Riordain, R., Moloney, E., Osullivan, K., & McCreary, C. (2010). Burning mouth syndrome and oral health-related quality of life: Is there a change over time? *Oral Diseases, 16*(7), 643–647. http://doi.org/10.1111/j.1601-0825.2010.01666.x

Savage, N. W., Boras, V. V, & Barker, K. (2006). Burning mouth syndrome: clinical presentation, diagnosis and treatment. *The Australasian Journal of Dermatology, 47*(2), 77–81; quiz 82–83. http://doi.org/10.1111/j.1440-0960.2006.00236.x

Spanemberg, J. C., Cherubini, K., De Figueiredo, M. A. Z., Yurgel, L. S., & Salum, F. G. (2012). Aetiology and therapeutics of burning mouth syndrome: An update. *Gerodontology.* http://doi.org/10.1111/j.1741-2358.2010.00384.x

Speciali, J. G., & Stuginski-Barbosa, J. (2008). Burning mouth syndrome. *Current Pain and Headache Reports.* http://doi.org/10.1007/s11916-008-0047-9

Stuginski-Barbosa, J., Rodrigues, G. G. R., Bigal, M. E., & Speciali, J. G. (2008). Burning mouth syndrome responsive to pramipexol. *Journal of Headache and Pain, 9*(1), 43–45. http://doi.org/10.1007/s10194-008-0003-4

Sun, A., Wu, K.-M., Wang, Y.-P., Lin, H.-P., Chen, H.-M., & Chiang, C.-P. (2013). Burning mouth syndrome: a review and update. *Journal of Oral Pathology & Medicine : Official Publication of the International Association of Oral Pathologists and the American Academy of Oral Pathology, 42,* 649–55. http://doi.org/10.1111/jop.12101

Thoppay, J. R., De Rossi, S. S., & Ciarrocca, K. N. (2013). Burning mouth syndrome. *Dental Clinics of North America.* http://doi.org/10.1016/j.cden.2013.04.010

Torgerson, R. R. (2010). Burning mouth syndrome. *Dermatologic Therapy.* http://doi.org/10.1111/j.1529-8019.2010.01325.x

Wandeur, T., De Moura, S. A. B., De Medeiros, A. M. C., MacHado, M. A. N., De Azevedo Alanis, L. R., Grégio, A. M. T., … De Lima, A. A. S. (2011). Exfoliative cytology of the oral mucosa in burning mouth syndrome: A cytomorphological and cytomorphometric analysis. *Gerodontology, 28*(1), 44–48. http://doi.org/10.1111/j.1741-2358.2009.00319.x

Zur, E. (2012). Burning mouth syndrome: a discussion of a complex pathology. *International Journal of Pharmaceutical Compounding, 16*(3), 196–205. Retrieved from

http://www.ncbi.nlm.nih.gov/pubmed/23050296\nhttp://www.scopus.com/inw
eid=2-s2.0-84868250574&partnerID=tZOtx3y1

Burning Mouth Syndrome Internet Articles and Research

Burning Mouth Syndrome | Causes & Risk Factors. (2015). Retrieved on
January 22, 2015, from http://familydoctor.org/familydoctor/en/diseases-
conditions/burning-mouth-syndrome/causes-risk-factors.html.

Burning Mouth Syndrome: Causes and Treatment Options – 1. (2015).
Retrieved on January 22, 2015, from http://www.1800dentist.com/burning-
mouth-syndrome/.

Burning Mouth Syndrome. (2015). Retrieved on January 22, 2015, from
http://bjp.sagepub.com/content/5/4/12.refs.

Burning Mouth Syndrome. (2015). Retrieved on January 22, 2015, from
http://emedicine.medscape.com/article/1508869-overview.

Burning Mouth Syndrome. (2015). Retrieved on January 22, 2015, from
http://www.sharecare.com/health/burning-mouth-syndrome.

Burning mouth syndrome Symptoms. (2015). Retrieved on January 22, 2015,
from http://www.mayoclinic.org/diseases-conditions/burning-mouth-
syndrome/basics/symptoms/con-20029596.

Burning mouth syndrome. (2015). Retrieved on January 22, 2015, from
http://en.wikipedia.org/wiki/Burning_mouth_syndrome.

Burning mouth. (2015). Retrieved on January 22, 2015, from
http://www.rightdiagnosis.com/sym/burning_mouth.htm.

Diabetes Mellitus – A Risk Factor For Periodontal Disease. (2015).
Retrieved on January 22, 2015, from https://ispub.com/IJFP/9/1/8342.

Diabetes and Periodontal Infection: Making the Connection. (2015).
Retrieved on January 22, 2015, from
http://clinical.diabetesjournals.org/content/23/4/171.full.

How to Manage Burning Mouth Syndrome. (2015). Retrieved on January 22,
2015, from http://www.everydayhealth.com/dental-health/how-to-manage-
burning-mouth-syndrome.aspx.

MayoClinic.com Health Library. (2015). Retrieved on January 22, 2015,
from http://www.riversideonline.com/health_reference/dental-
care/ds00462.cfm.

Order Free Publications. (2015). Retrieved on January 22, 2015, from http://www.nidcr.nih.gov/AtoZ/LetterO/OrderPublications.htm.

Pharmacological treatment of burning mouth syndrome: A review .... (2015). Retrieved on January 22, 2015, from http://scielo.isciii.es/scielo.php?script=sci_arttext&pid=S1698-69462007000400007.

Problems in the Mouth. Free Medical Information | Patient.co.uk. (2015). Retrieved on January 22, 2015, from http://www.patient.co.uk/doctor/problems-in-the-mouth.

Related Diseases. (2015). Retrieved on January 22, 2015, from http://www.medicinenet.com/burning_mouth_syndrome/related-conditions/index.htm.

Sjogren's Syndrome Symptoms, Causes, Treatment. (2015). Retrieved on January 22, 2015, from http://www.medicinenet.com/sjogrens_syndrome/page2.htm.

Temporomandibular Disorders in Burning Mouth Syndrome Patients .... (2015). Retrieved on January 22, 2015, from http://www.medsci.org/v10p1784.htm.

Tongue Burn: Causes, Risk Factors & Symptoms. (2015). Retrieved on January 22, 2015, from http://www.healthline.com/health/tongue-burn.

Advanced Dental Specialists. (2015). *The Mouth*. Retrieved on January 22, 2015, from http://advanceddentalspecialists.com/YourHealth/TheMouthBodyConnection.

Grushka M , et al.. (2015). *Burning mouth syndrome..* Retrieved on January 22, 2015, from http://www.ncbi.nlm.nih.gov/pubmed/11871678.

XOOPS. (2015). *UCLA Department of Medicine*. Retrieved on January 22, 2015, from http://www.med.ucla.edu/modules/wfsection/article.php?articleid=266.

CHAPTER 5

SYMPTOMS

&

SIGNS

Distinguishing Symtoms from Signs

According to the National Institutes of Health, a symptom is a "physical or mental problem that a person experiences that may indicate a disease or condition." While a sign can mean the same thing noteworthy to the definition of symptom is that symptoms are typically *not* seen **(observed)** by other people and generally can *not* be independently identified **(for diagnosis)** by doctors using medical tests. Signs, on the other hand, can be both **observed** and used to independently **diagnosis** a condition without patient input. Therefore, while the presence or absence of a symptom can not conclusively be used to determine the presence or absence of disease, a sign can be, or cynically speaking, a patient can claim nonexistent symptoms that can not be refuted by doctors but signs can be identified and measured independent of patient input. Common symptoms for many health conditions include fatigue, pain, nausea, and headache. On the other hand, signs of disease often include skin rashes, sweating, uncontrollable bleeding, and difficulties with speech. Notwithstanding "provability," both the accurate portrayl of symptoms and observable signs are critical in disease diagnosis, treatment, and management.

Types of Symptoms

Symptoms of disease can be characterized in a number of ways. First, they can be described by their presence or absence. In this regard, symptoms may be persistent or long-lasting **(chronic)**, ebb and flow at regular or irregular intervals **(relapsing)**, or disappear completely even though the underlying disease may still be present **(remitting)**. Further, some diseases may be **asymptomatic** meaning the underlying disease condition presents no symptoms whatsoever. Frequently, conditions like diabetes and high blood pressure are asymptomatic in that they can be present with no symptoms.

Symptoms can also be classified by the way they impact the "total person." In describing mental disorders in particular, symptoms can be described as **positive** or **negative**. Many people mistakenly imply positive and negative symptoms to mean good and bad symptoms. Instead, positive and negative symptoms should be considered in a more mathematical plus or minus sense. Thus, positive symptoms are feelings (stimulus) in addition to or added to a person's normal spectrum of feelings/stimulus and negative symptoms are feelings/stimulus taken away from the normal spectrum. Therefore, for a mental health disorder like schizophrenia a positive symptom may include hallucinations where a person sees things in addition to things actually present. Conversely, a negative symptom may include a "flat affect" where facial expressions and typical speaking rhythms and changes in tone found in a normal person are absent in a person with Burning Mouth Syndrome. Other negative symptoms commonly found in patients with mental health illnesses include taking *less* pleasure in life, speaking *less*, or engaging in *fewer* activities all when compared to persons without mental illness.

Burning Mouth Syndrome Journal Articles

Balasubramaniam, R., Klasser, G. D., & Delcanho, R. (2009). Separating oral burning from burning mouth syndrome: Unravelling a diagnostic enigma. *Australian Dental Journal*. http://doi.org/10.1111/j.1834-7819.2009.01153.x

Barker, K. E., Batstone, M. D., & Savage, N. W. (2009). Comparison of treatment modalities in burning mouth syndrome. *Australian Dental Journal*, *54*(4), 300–305. http://doi.org/10.1111/j.1834-7819.2009.01154.x

Barker, K. E., & Savage, N. W. (2005). Burning mouth syndrome: An update on recent findings. *Australian Dental Journal*. http://doi.org/10.1111/j.1834-7819.2005.tb00363.x

Brailo, V., Vuéiaeeviae-Boras, V., Alajbeg, I. Z., Alajbeg, I., Lukenda, J., & Aeurkoviae, M. (2006). Oral burning symptoms and burning mouth syndrome-significance of different variables in 150 patients. *Medicina Oral, Patología Oral Y Cirugía Bucal.*, *11*(3).

Brufau-Redondo, C., Martín-Brufau, R., Corbalán-Velez, R., & De Concepción-Salesa, a. (2002). Burning mouth syndrome. *British Dental Journal*, *45*(6), 237–241. http://doi.org/10.1111/j.1526-4637.2010.01035.x

Buljan, D., Savic, I., & Karlovic, D. (2008). CORRELATION BETWEEN ANXIETY, DEPRESSION AND BURNING MOUTH SYNDROME. *ACTA CLINICA CROATICA*, *47*(4), 211–216.

Cerchiari, D. P., de Moricz, R. D., Sanjar, F. A., Rapoport, P. B., Moretti, G., & Guerra, M. M. (2006). Burning mouth syndrome: etiology. *Brazilian Journal of Otorhinolaryngology*, *72*(3), 419–23. http://doi.org/S0034-72992006000300021 [pii]

Cibirka, R. M., Nelson, S. K., & Lefebvre, C. A. (1999). A review of burning mouth syndrome. *The Journal of Prosthetic Dentistry*, *78*(1), 29–35.

Coon, E. A., & Laughlin, R. S. (2012). Burning mouth syndrome in Parkinson's disease: Dopamine as cure or cause? *Journal of Headache and Pain*, *13*(3), 255–257. http://doi.org/10.1007/s10194-012-0421-1

Crow, H. C., & Gonzalez, Y. (2012). Burning Mouth Syndrome. *Oral and Maxillofacial Surgery Clinics of North America*, *65*(5), 343–347. http://doi.org/10.4248/IJOS10008

Crow, H. C., & Gonzalez, Y. (2013). Burning Mouth Syndrome. *Oral and Maxillofacial Surgery Clinics of North America*.

http://doi.org/10.1016/j.coms.2012.11.001

Culhane, N. S., & Hodle, A. D. (2001). Burning mouth syndrome after taking clonazepam. *Annals of Pharmacotherapy, 35*(7-8), 874–876. http://doi.org/10.1345/aph.1Z434

Dahiya, P., Kamal, R., Kumar, M., Niti, Gupta, R., & Chaudhary, K. (2013). Burning mouth syndrome and menopause. *International Journal of Preventive Medicine, 4*(1), 15–20.

De Moraes, M., do Amaral Bezerra, B. A., da Rocha Neto, P. C., de Oliveira Soares, A. C. A., Pinto, L. P., & de Lisboa Lopes Costa, A. (2012). Randomized trials for the treatment of burning mouth syndrome: an evidence-based review of the literature. *Journal of Oral Pathology & Medicine : Official Publication of the International Association of Oral Pathologists and the American Academy of Oral Pathology, 41*(4), 281–7. http://doi.org/10.1111/j.1600-0714.2011.01100.x

De Souza, F. T. A., Amaral, T. M. P., Dos Santos, T. P. M., Abdo, E. N., Aguiar, M. C. F., Teixeira, A. L., … Silva, T. A. (2012). Burning mouth syndrome: A therapeutic approach involving mechanical salivary stimulation. *Headache, 52*(6), 1026–1034. http://doi.org/10.1111/j.1526-4610.2011.02037.x

Drage, L. A., & Rogers, R. S. 3rd. (2003). Burning mouth syndrome. *Dermatologic Clinics*. Retrieved from http://ovidsp.ovid.com/ovidweb.cgi?T=JS&PAGE=reference&D=med4&NEWS=N&AN=12622276

Friedman, D. I. (2010). Topirimate-induced burning mouth syndrome. *Headache, 50*(8), 1383–1385. http://doi.org/10.1111/j.1526-4610.2010.01720.x

Grushka, M., Epstein, J. B., & Gorsky, M. (2002a). Burning mouth syndrome. *American Family Physician, 65*(4). http://doi.org/10.3748/wjg.v19.i5.665

Grushka, M., Epstein, J. B., & Gorsky, M. (2002). Burning mouth syndrome. *Am Fam Physician, 65*(4), 615–620. Retrieved from http://www.ncbi.nlm.nih.gov/entrez/query.fcgi?cmd=Retrieve&db=PubMed&dopt=Citation&list_uids=11871678

Grushka, M., Epstein, J., & Gorsky, M. (2002b). Burning mouth syndrome. *American Family Physician, 65*(4), 615–620. Retrieved from http://www.ncbi.nlm.nih.gov/pubmed/11871678

Gurvits, G. E., & Tan, A. (2013). Burning mouth syndrome. *World Journal of Gastroenterology : WJG, 19*(5), 665–72. http://doi.org/10.3748/wjg.v19.i5.665

Klasser, G. D., Epstein, J. B., & Villines, D. (2011). Management of burning mouth syndrome. *Journal (Canadian Dental Association), 77*, b151. Retrieved from http://www.ncbi.nlm.nih.gov/pubmed/22260804

Klasser, G. D., Fischer, D. J., & Epstein, J. B. (2008a). Burning Mouth Syndrome: Recognition, Understanding, and Management. *Oral and Maxillofacial Surgery Clinics of North America.* http://doi.org/10.1016/j.coms.2007.12.012

Klasser, G. D., Fischer, D. J., & Epstein, J. B. (2008b). Burning mouth syndrome: recognition, understanding, and management. *Oral Maxillofacial Surg Clin N Am, 20*(2), 255–71, vii. http://doi.org/10.1016/j.coms.2007.12.012

Lamey, P.-J., Freeman, R., Eddie, S.-A., Pankhurst, C., & Rees, T. (2005). Vulnerability and presenting symptoms in burning mouth syndrome. *Oral Surgery, Oral Medicine, Oral Pathology, Oral Radiology, and Endodontics, 99*(1), 48–54. http://doi.org/10.1016/j.tripleo.2004.01.021

Lauria, G., Majorana, A., Borgna, M., Lombardi, R., Penza, P., Padovani, A., & Sapelli, P. (2005). Trigeminal small-fiber sensory neuropathy causes burning mouth syndrome. *Pain, 115*(3), 332–337. http://doi.org/10.1016/j.pain.2005.03.028

López-Jornet, P., Camacho-Alonso, F., & Andujar-Mateos, P. (2011). A prospective, randomized study on the efficacy of tongue protector in patients with burning mouth syndrome. *Oral Diseases, 17*(3), 277–282. http://doi.org/10.1111/j.1601-0825.2010.01737.x

López-Jornet, P., Camacho-Alonso, F., Andujar-Mateos, P., Sánchez-Siles, M., & Gómez-Garcia, F. (2010). Burning mouth syndrome: an update. *Medicina Oral, Patología Oral Y Cirugía Bucal, 15*(4), e562–8. Retrieved from http://www.ncbi.nlm.nih.gov/pubmed/23772971

Marino, R., Capaccio, P., Pignataro, L., & Spadari, F. (2009). Burning mouth syndrome: The role of contact hypersensitivity. *Oral Diseases, 15*(4), 255–258. http://doi.org/10.1111/j.1601-0825.2009.01515.x

Mignogna, M. D., Pollio, A., Fortuna, G., Leuci, S., Ruoppo, E., Adamo, D., & Zarrelli, C. (2011). Unexplained somatic comorbidities in patients with burning mouth syndrome: a controlled clinical study. *Journal of Orofacial Pain, 25*(2), 131–140.

Mínguez Serra, M. P., Salort Llorca, C., & Silvestre Donat, F. J. (2007). Pharmacological treatment of burning mouth syndrome: A review and update. *Medicina Oral, Patología Oral Y Cirugía Bucal.*

Minor, J. S., & Epstein, J. B. (2011a). Burning mouth syndrome and secondary oral burning. *Otolaryngologic Clinics of North America.* http://doi.org/10.1016/j.otc.2010.09.008

Minor, J. S., & Epstein, J. B. (2011b). Burning mouth syndrome and secondary oral burning. *Otolaryngol Clin N Am, 44*(1), 205–19, vii. http://doi.org/10.1016/j.otc.2010.09.008

Mock, D., & Chugh, D. (2010). Burning mouth syndrome. *International Journal of Oral Science, 2*(1), 1–4. http://doi.org/10.4248/IJOS10008

Muzyka, B. C., & De Rossi, S. S. (1999). A review of burning mouth syndrome. *Cutis; Cutaneous Medicine for the Practitioner, 64*(1), 29–35.

Ni Riordain, R., Moloney, E., Osullivan, K., & McCreary, C. (2010). Burning mouth syndrome and oral health-related quality of life: Is there a change over time? *Oral Diseases, 16*(7), 643–647. http://doi.org/10.1111/j.1601-0825.2010.01666.x

Rhodus, N. L., Carlson, C. R., & Miller, C. S. (2003). Burning mouth (syndrome) disorder. *Quintessence International (Berlin, Germany : 1985), 34*(8), 587–593.

Sardella, A., Lodi, G., Demarosi, F., Bez, C., Cassano, S., & Carrassi, A. (2006). Burning mouth syndrome: A retrospective study investigating spontaneous remission and response to treatments. *Oral Diseases.* http://doi.org/10.1111/j.1601-0825.2005.01174.x

Savage, N. W., Boras, V. V, & Barker, K. (2006). Burning mouth syndrome: clinical presentation, diagnosis and treatment. *The Australasian Journal of Dermatology, 47*(2), 77–81; quiz 82–83. http://doi.org/10.1111/j.1440-0960.2006.00236.x

Ship, J. A., Grushka, M., Lipton, J. A., Mott, A. E., Sessle, B. J., & Dionne, R. A. (1995). Burning mouth syndrome: an update. *Journal of the American Dental Association (1939), 126*(7), 842–853.

Silvestre, F. J., Silvestre-Rangil, J., Tamarit-Santafé, C., & Bautista, D.

(2012). Application of a capsaicin rinse in the treatment of burning mouth syndrome. *Medicina Oral, Patologia Oral Y Cirugia Bucal, 17*(1). http://doi.org/10.4317/medoral.17219

Spanemberg, J. C., Cherubini, K., De Figueiredo, M. A. Z., Yurgel, L. S., & Salum, F. G. (2012). Aetiology and therapeutics of burning mouth syndrome: An update. *Gerodontology*. http://doi.org/10.1111/j.1741-2358.2010.00384.x

Speciali, J. G., & Stuginski-Barbosa, J. (2008). Burning mouth syndrome. *Current Pain and Headache Reports*. http://doi.org/10.1007/s11916-008-0047-9

Stuginski-Barbosa, J., Rodrigues, G. G. R., Bigal, M. E., & Speciali, J. G. (2008). Burning mouth syndrome responsive to pramipexol. *Journal of Headache and Pain*, 9(1), 43–45. http://doi.org/10.1007/s10194-008-0003-4

Sun, A., Wu, K.-M., Wang, Y.-P., Lin, H.-P., Chen, H.-M., & Chiang, C.-P. (2013). Burning mouth syndrome: a review and update. *Journal of Oral Pathology & Medicine : Official Publication of the International Association of Oral Pathologists and the American Academy of Oral Pathology*, 42, 649–55. http://doi.org/10.1111/jop.12101

Thoppay, J. R., De Rossi, S. S., & Ciarrocca, K. N. (2013). Burning mouth syndrome. *Dental Clinics of North America*. http://doi.org/10.1016/j.cden.2013.04.010

Torgerson, R. R. (2010). Burning mouth syndrome. *Dermatologic Therapy*. http://doi.org/10.1111/j.1529-8019.2010.01325.x

Varvat, J., Thomas-Anterion, C., Decousus, M., Perret-Liaudet, A., & Laurent, B. Atypical Lewy body disease revealed by burning mouth syndrome and a pseudo-psychiatric syndrome, 166 Revue neurologique 547–549 (2010). http://doi.org/10.1016/j.neurol.2009.10.018

Zakrzewska, J. M., Forssell, H., & Glenny, A.-M. (2003). Interventions for the treatment of burning mouth syndrome: a systematic review. *Journal of Orofacial Pain*, *17*(4), 293–300.

Zur, E. (2012). Burning mouth syndrome: a discussion of a complex pathology. *International Journal of Pharmaceutical Compounding*, *16*(3), 196–205. Retrieved from http://www.ncbi.nlm.nih.gov/pubmed/23050296\nhttp://www.scopus.com/inward/record.url?eid=2-s2.0-84868250574&partnerID=tZOtx3y1

Burning Mouth Syndrome Internet Articles and Research

9 Oral Symptoms You Shouldn't Ignore. (2015). Retrieved on January 22, 2015, from http://www.everydayhealth.com/dental-health-pictures/icky-mouth-mysteries-solved.aspx.

Bruxism: Signs And Symptoms. (2015). Retrieved on January 22, 2015, from http://www.colgateprofessional.com/patient-education/articles/bruxism-signs-and-symptoms.

Burning Mouth Syndrome | Overview. (2015). Retrieved on January 22, 2015, from http://familydoctor.org/familydoctor/en/diseases-conditions/burning-mouth-syndrome.html.

Burning Mouth Syndrome: Causes and Treatment Options – 1. (2015). Retrieved on January 22, 2015, from http://www.1800dentist.com/burning-mouth-syndrome/.

Burning Mouth Syndrome: Learn About Symptoms. (2015). Retrieved on January 22, 2015, from http://www.medicinenet.com/burning_mouth_syndrome/article.htm.

Burning Mouth Syndrome. (2015). Retrieved on January 22, 2015, from http://emedicine.medscape.com/article/1508869-overview.

Burning Mouth Syndrome. (2015). Retrieved on January 22, 2015, from http://www.aafp.org/afp/2002/0215/p615.html.

Burning Mouth Syndrome. (2015). Retrieved on January 22, 2015, from http://www.colgateprofessional.com/patient-education/articles/burning-mouth-syndrome.

Burning Mouth Syndrome. (2015). Retrieved on January 22, 2015, from http://www.dentalgentlecare.com/burning_mouth_syndrome.htm.

Burning Mouth Syndrome. (2015). Retrieved on January 22, 2015, from http://www.nidcr.nih.gov/oralhealth/Topics/Burning/BurningMouthSyndrome

Burning Mouth Syndrome. (2015). Retrieved on January 22, 2015, from http://www.sharecare.com/health/burning-mouth-syndrome.

Burning Mouth Syndrome. (2015). Retrieved on January 22, 2015, from http://www.webmd.com/oral-health/burning-mouth-syndrome.

Burning Mouth Syndrome. (2015). Retrieved on January 22, 2015, from http://www.yourdentistryguide.com/burning-mouth/.

Burning Tongue | 34. (2015). Retrieved on January 22, 2015, from http://www.34-menopause-symptoms.com/burning-tongue.htm.

Burning mouth syndrome Symptoms. (2015). Retrieved on January 22, 2015, from http://www.mayoclinic.org/diseases-conditions/burning-mouth-syndrome/basics/symptoms/con-20029596.

Burning mouth syndrome. DermNet NZ. (2015). Retrieved on January 22, 2015, from http://www.dermnetnz.org/site-age-specific/burning-mouth.html.

Burning mouth syndrome. (2015). Retrieved on January 22, 2015, from http://en.wikipedia.org/wiki/Burning_mouth_syndrome.

Burning mouth syndrome. (2015). Retrieved on January 22, 2015, from http://www.webmd.boots.com/oral-health/burning-mouth-syndrome.

Mouth Sores and Inflammation: Symptoms of Oral and Dental .... (2015). Retrieved on January 22, 2015, from http://www.merckmanuals.com/home/mouth_and_dental_disorders/symptoms

Natural Cures for Burning Mouth Syndrome. (2015). Retrieved on January 22, 2015, from http://www.earthclinic.com/cures/burning-mouth-syndrome.html.

Tongue Burn: Causes, Risk Factors & Symptoms. (2015). Retrieved on January 22, 2015, from http://www.healthline.com/health/tongue-burn.

Nick Senzee. (2015). *Burning Mouth Syndrome.* Retrieved on January 22, 2015, from http://www.aaom.com/index.php?option=com_content&view=article&id=81:burning-mouth-syndrome&catid=22:patient-condition-information&Itemid=120.

Zakrzewska JM , et al.. (2015). *Interventions for the treatment of burning mouth syndrome..* Retrieved on January 22, 2015, from http://www.ncbi.nlm.nih.gov/pubmed/11687027.

CHAPTER 6

DIAGNOSIS

This Chapter will discuss the concept of diagnosis, including the difference between health conditions that are **misdiagnosed** and those that are **undiagnosed**. This Chapter will also examine the difference between common diagnosis and a differential diagnoses.

The Diagnostic and Differential Diagnostic Process

The term diagnosis refers to the *process* of identifying a disease, based on the signs and symptoms of disease, and a **diagnostic procedure** is a method used to arrive at a diagnosis. Most frequently, doctors base diagnostic determinations on **medical tests** and **observation** to identify a disease or condition. Through test and observation the doctor is attempting to either identify a physical, biological, chemical, emotional, or psychological condition not normally present in a healthy person **OR** one that is present in a healthy person but absent in a person with a particular illness or disease. In this regard, the diagnostic process generally begins with the doctor making an educated guess as to which condition is most likely present, and through tests and observation confirming or denying the presence or absence of disease or illness.

When a doctor fails to diagnosis a disease that is actually present the disease has gone **undiagnosed** and when the doctor determines one disease is present when in fact it is another the health condition is **misdiagnosed**. Obviously, both concepts can go hand-in-hand as the the disease that is present but not identified is undiagnosed and the disease that is identified but not present is misdiagnosed.

On the other hand, a process of **differential diagnosis** is one that, based on the signs and symptoms, a doctor determines that two or more alternative diseases or conditions are nearly equally likely to be present. In essence, the differential diagnostic procedure is a "process of elimination" where a list of possible diseases and disorders is constructed, and possible diseases are removed one-by-one. To eliminate alternative health problems, a physician will use a combination of medical tests, observation, intuition, and past experience to rule-out individual health conditions until only a single condition remains on the list. Because a differential diagnosis attempts to distinguish health disorders that present themselves in a very similar manner, the differential diagnostic process is typically more involved and time-consuming than normal diagnostic protocols. For the same reason and for some conditions, the differential diagnostic process may result in fewer instances of undiagnosed disease but more instances of misdiagnosis.

Medical tests are used to screen for or diagnose health conditions that may be present in a patient or monitor conditions that already exist. **Diagnostic tests** are generally performed only after a patient reports symptoms of a disease or health condition or in response to signs observed by a medical professional. The most methods to diagnose Burning Mouth Syndrome are discussed below.

Burning Mouth Syndrome Journal Articles

Abetz, L. M., & Savage, N. W. (2009). Burning mouth syndrome and psychological disorders. *Australian Dental Journal, 54*(2), 84–93; quiz 173. http://doi.org/10.1111/j.1834-7819.2009.01099.x

Balasubramaniam, R., Klasser, G. D., & Delcanho, R. (2009). Separating oral burning from burning mouth syndrome: Unravelling a diagnostic enigma. *Australian Dental Journal.* http://doi.org/10.1111/j.1834-7819.2009.01153.x

Barker, K. E., & Savage, N. W. (2005). Burning mouth syndrome: An update on recent findings. *Australian Dental Journal.* http://doi.org/10.1111/j.1834-7819.2005.tb00363.x

Boy-Metin, Z., Kayhan, K. B., & Unür, M. (2008). Burning mouth syndrome. *Kulak Burun Boğaz Ihtisas Dergisi : KBB = Journal of Ear, Nose, and Throat, 18*(3), 188–96. Retrieved from http://www.ncbi.nlm.nih.gov/pubmed/19388467

Brufau-Redondo, C., Martín-Brufau, R., Corbalán-Velez, R., & De Concepción-Salesa, a. (2002). Burning mouth syndrome. *British Dental Journal, 45*(6), 237–241. http://doi.org/10.1111/j.1526-4637.2010.01035.x

Brufau-Redondo, C., Martin-Brufau, R., Corbalan-Velez, R., & de Concepcion-Salesa, A. (2008). {[}Burning mouth syndrome{]}. *Actas Dermosifiliogr, 99*(6), 431–440.

Cerchiari, D. P., de Moricz, R. D., Sanjar, F. A., Rapoport, P. B., Moretti, G., & Guerra, M. M. (2006). Burning mouth syndrome: etiology. *Brazilian Journal of Otorhinolaryngology, 72*(3), 419–23. http://doi.org/S0034-72992006000300021 [pii]

Coon, E. A., & Laughlin, R. S. (2012). Burning mouth syndrome in Parkinson's disease: Dopamine as cure or cause? *Journal of Headache and Pain, 13*(3), 255–257. http://doi.org/10.1007/s10194-012-0421-1

Crow, H. C., & Gonzalez, Y. (2012). Burning Mouth Syndrome. *Oral and Maxillofacial Surgery Clinics of North America, 65*(5), 343–347. http://doi.org/10.4248/IJOS10008

Crow, H. C., & Gonzalez, Y. (2013). Burning Mouth Syndrome. *Oral and Maxillofacial Surgery Clinics of North America.* http://doi.org/10.1016/j.coms.2012.11.001

De Moraes, M., do Amaral Bezerra, B. A., da Rocha Neto, P. C., de Oliveira

Soares, A. C. A., Pinto, L. P., & de Lisboa Lopes Costa, A. (2012). Randomized trials for the treatment of burning mouth syndrome: an evidence-based review of the literature. *Journal of Oral Pathology & Medicine : Official Publication of the International Association of Oral Pathologists and the American Academy of Oral Pathology, 41*(4), 281–7. http://doi.org/10.1111/j.1600-0714.2011.01100.x

Ducasse, D., Courtet, P., & Olie, E. (2013). Burning mouth syndrome: current clinical, physiopathologic, and therapeutic data. *Regional Anesthesia and Pain Medicine, 38*(5), 380–90. http://doi.org/10.1097/AAP.0b013e3182a1f0db

Fedele, S., Fricchione, G., Porter, & Mignogna, M. (2007a). Stomatodynia or burning mouth syndrome. *Acta Dermatovenerologica Croatica ADC Hrvatsko Dermatolosko Drustvo, 100*(4), 231–235. Retrieved from http://discovery.ucl.ac.uk/148057/

Fedele, S., Fricchione, G., Porter, S. R., & Mignogna, M. D. (2007b). Stomatodynia or burning mouth syndrome. *Acta Dermatovenerologica Croatica ADC Hrvatsko Dermatolosko Drustvo, 11*(4), 231–235. Retrieved from http://discovery.ucl.ac.uk/148057/

Friedman, D. I. (2010). Topirimate-induced burning mouth syndrome. *Headache, 50*(8), 1383–1385. http://doi.org/10.1111/j.1526-4610.2010.01720.x

Gerlinger, I. (2012). [Burning sensation in oral cavity--burning mouth syndrome in everyday medical practice]. *Ideggyógyászati Szemle, 65*(9-10), 295–301. Retrieved from http://www.ncbi.nlm.nih.gov/pubmed/23126213

Grushka, M., Epstein, J. B., & Gorsky, M. (2002). Burning mouth syndrome. *American Family Physician, 65*(4). http://doi.org/10.3748/wjg.v19.i5.665

Gurvits, G. E., & Tan, A. (2013). Burning mouth syndrome. *World Journal of Gastroenterology : WJG, 19*(5), 665–72. http://doi.org/10.3748/wjg.v19.i5.665

Jääskeläinen, S. K. (2012). Pathophysiology of primary burning mouth syndrome. *Clinical Neurophysiology.* http://doi.org/10.1016/j.clinph.2011.07.054

Jacobson, A. (2006). The diagnosis of burning mouth syndrome represents a challenge for clinicians. *American Journal of Orthodontics and Dentofacial Orthopedics.* http://doi.org/10.1016/j.ajodo.2005.08.021

Javali, M. A. (2013). Burning mouth syndrome: An enigmatic disorder. *Kathmandu University Medical Journal.*

Klasser, G. D., Epstein, J. B., & Villines, D. (2011). Management of burning mouth syndrome. *Journal (Canadian Dental Association), 77,* b151. Retrieved from http://www.ncbi.nlm.nih.gov/pubmed/22260804

Klasser, G. D., Epstein, J. B., & Villines, D. (2012). Management of burning mouth syndrome. *The Journal of the Michigan Dental Association, 94*(6), 43–6. Retrieved from http://www.pubmedcentral.nih.gov/articlerender.fcgi?artid=3860198&tool=pmcentrez&rendertype=abstract

Klasser, G. D., Fischer, D. J., & Epstein, J. B. (2008a). Burning Mouth Syndrome: Recognition, Understanding, and Management. *Oral and Maxillofacial Surgery Clinics of North America.* http://doi.org/10.1016/j.coms.2007.12.012

Klasser, G. D., Fischer, D. J., & Epstein, J. B. (2008b). Burning mouth syndrome: recognition, understanding, and management. *Oral Maxillofacial Surg Clin N Am, 20*(2), 255–71, vii. http://doi.org/10.1016/j.coms.2007.12.012

Lauria, G., Majorana, A., Borgna, M., Lombardi, R., Penza, P., Padovani, A., & Sapelli, P. (2005). Trigeminal small-fiber sensory neuropathy causes burning mouth syndrome. *Pain, 115*(3), 332–337. http://doi.org/10.1016/j.pain.2005.03.028

López-Jornet, P., Camacho-Alonso, F., & Andujar-Mateos, P. (2011). A prospective, randomized study on the efficacy of tongue protector in patients with burning mouth syndrome. *Oral Diseases, 17*(3), 277–282. http://doi.org/10.1111/j.1601-0825.2010.01737.x

López-Jornet, P., Camacho-Alonso, F., Andujar-Mateos, P., Sánchez-Siles, M., & Gómez-Garcia, F. (2010). Burning mouth syndrome: an update. *Medicina Oral, Patología Oral Y Cirugía Bucal, 15*(4), e562–8. Retrieved from http://www.ncbi.nlm.nih.gov/pubmed/23772971

Maltsman-Tseikhin, A., Moricca, P., & Niv, D. (2007). Burning mouth syndrome: will better understanding yield better management? *Pain Practice : The Official Journal of World Institute of Pain, 7*(2), 151–162. http://doi.org/10.1111/j.1533-2500.2007.00124.x

Marino, R., Capaccio, P., Pignataro, L., & Spadari, F. (2009). Burning mouth syndrome: The role of contact hypersensitivity. *Oral Diseases, 15*(4), 255–

258. http://doi.org/10.1111/j.1601-0825.2009.01515.x

Minor, J. S., & Epstein, J. B. (2011a). Burning mouth syndrome and secondary oral burning. *Otolaryngologic Clinics of North America.* http://doi.org/10.1016/j.otc.2010.09.008

Minor, J. S., & Epstein, J. B. (2011b). Burning mouth syndrome and secondary oral burning. *Otolaryngol Clin N Am, 44*(1), 205–19, vii. http://doi.org/10.1016/j.otc.2010.09.008

Mock, D., & Chugh, D. (2010). Burning mouth syndrome. *Int.J.Oral Sci., 2*(1), 1–4.

Mock, D., & Chugh, D. (2010). Burning mouth syndrome. *International Journal of Oral Science, 2*(1), 1–4. http://doi.org/10.4248/IJOS10008

Ni Riordain, R., Moloney, E., Osullivan, K., & McCreary, C. (2010). Burning mouth syndrome and oral health-related quality of life: Is there a change over time? *Oral Diseases, 16*(7), 643–647. http://doi.org/10.1111/j.1601-0825.2010.01666.x

Pinto, A., Stoopler, E. T., DeRossi, S. S., Sollecito, T. P., & Popovic, R. (2002). Burning mouth syndrome: a guide for the general practitioner. *General Dentistry, 51*(5), 458–61; quiz 462. Retrieved from http://www.ncbi.nlm.nih.gov/pubmed/15055637

Rhodus, N. L., Carlson, C. R., & Miller, C. S. (2003). Burning mouth (syndrome) disorder. *Quintessence International (Berlin, Germany : 1985), 34*(8), 587–593.

Salort Llorca, C., Mínguez Serra, M. P., & Silvestre, F. J. (2008). Drug-induced burning mouth syndrome: A new etiological diagnosis. *Medicina Oral, Patologia Oral Y Cirugia Bucal, 13*(3), 167–170. http://doi.org/10488787 [pii]

Savage, N. W. (1996). Burning mouth syndrome: patient management. *Australian Dental Journal, 41*(6), 363–366.

Savage, N. W., Boras, V. V, & Barker, K. (2006). Burning mouth syndrome: clinical presentation, diagnosis and treatment. *The Australasian Journal of Dermatology, 47*(2), 77–81; quiz 82–83. http://doi.org/10.1111/j.1440-0960.2006.00236.x

Spanemberg, J. C., Cherubini, K., De Figueiredo, M. A. Z., Yurgel, L. S., & Salum, F. G. (2012). Aetiology and therapeutics of burning mouth syndrome:

An update. *Gerodontology*. http://doi.org/10.1111/j.1741-2358.2010.00384.x

Speciali, J. G., & Stuginski-Barbosa, J. (2008). Burning mouth syndrome. *Current Pain and Headache Reports*. http://doi.org/10.1007/s11916-008-0047-9

Speciali, J. G., & Stuginski-Barbosa, J. (2008). Burning mouth syndrome. *Curr Pain Headache Rep., 12*(4), 279–284.

Stuginski-Barbosa, J., Rodrigues, G. G. R., Bigal, M. E., & Speciali, J. G. (2008). Burning mouth syndrome responsive to pramipexol. *Journal of Headache and Pain, 9*(1), 43–45. http://doi.org/10.1007/s10194-008-0003-4

Sun, A., Wu, K.-M., Wang, Y.-P., Lin, H.-P., Chen, H.-M., & Chiang, C.-P. (2013). Burning mouth syndrome: a review and update. *Journal of Oral Pathology & Medicine : Official Publication of the International Association of Oral Pathologists and the American Academy of Oral Pathology, 42*, 649–55. http://doi.org/10.1111/jop.12101

Thoppay, J. R., De Rossi, S. S., & Ciarrocca, K. N. (2013). Burning mouth syndrome. *Dental Clinics of North America*. http://doi.org/10.1016/j.cden.2013.04.010

Torgerson, R. R. (2010). Burning mouth syndrome. *Dermatologic Therapy*. http://doi.org/10.1111/j.1529-8019.2010.01325.x

Varvat, J., Thomas-Anterion, C., Decousus, M., Perret-Liaudet, A., & Laurent, B. Atypical Lewy body disease revealed by burning mouth syndrome and a pseudo-psychiatric syndrome, 166 Revue neurologique 547–549 (2010). http://doi.org/10.1016/j.neurol.2009.10.018

Witt, E., & Palla, S. (2002). Mundbrennen, [Burning mouth]. *Schmerz (Berlin, Germany), 16*(5), 389–94. http://doi.org/10.1007/s00482-002-0149-y

Zur, E. (2012). Burning mouth syndrome: a discussion of a complex pathology. *International Journal of Pharmaceutical Compounding, 16*(3), 196–205. Retrieved from http://www.ncbi.nlm.nih.gov/pubmed/23050296\nhttp://www.scopus.com/inw eid=2-s2.0-84868250574&partnerID=tZOtx3y1

Burning Mouth Syndrome Internet Articles and Research

Bruxism: Signs And Symptoms. (2015). Retrieved on January 22, 2015, from http://www.colgateprofessional.com/patient-education/articles/bruxism-signs-and-symptoms.

Burning Mouth Syndrome is often difficult to diagnose. (2015). Retrieved on January 22, 2015, from http://www.sciencedaily.com/releases/2013/10/131023100957.htm.

Burning Mouth Syndrome | Overview. (2015). Retrieved on January 22, 2015, from http://familydoctor.org/familydoctor/en/diseases-conditions/burning-mouth-syndrome.html.

Burning Mouth Syndrome: Causes and Treatment Options – 1. (2015). Retrieved on January 22, 2015, from http://www.1800dentist.com/burning-mouth-syndrome/.

Burning Mouth Syndrome: Learn About Symptoms. (2015). Retrieved on January 22, 2015, from http://www.medicinenet.com/burning_mouth_syndrome/article.htm.

Burning Mouth Syndrome. (2015). Retrieved on January 22, 2015, from http://emedicine.medscape.com/article/1508869-overview.

Burning Mouth Syndrome. (2015). Retrieved on January 22, 2015, from http://www.aafp.org/afp/2002/0215/p615.html.

Burning Mouth Syndrome. (2015). Retrieved on January 22, 2015, from http://www.dentalgentlecare.com/burning_mouth_syndrome.htm.

Burning Mouth Syndrome. (2015). Retrieved on January 22, 2015, from http://www.nidcr.nih.gov/oralhealth/Topics/Burning/BurningMouthSyndrome

Burning Mouth Syndrome. (2015). Retrieved on January 22, 2015, from http://www.sharecare.com/health/burning-mouth-syndrome.

Burning Mouth Syndrome. (2015). Retrieved on January 22, 2015, from http://www.webmd.com/oral-health/burning-mouth-syndrome.

Burning Mouth Syndrome. (2015). Retrieved on January 22, 2015, from http://www.yourdentistryguide.com/burning-mouth/.

Burning Mouth. (2015). Retrieved on January 22, 2015, from http://my.clevelandclinic.org/health/diseases_conditions/hic_burning_mouth.

Burning Tongue | 34. (2015). Retrieved on January 22, 2015, from http://www.34-menopause-symptoms.com/burning-tongue.htm.

Burning mouth syndrome Symptoms. (2015). Retrieved on January 22, 2015, from http://www.mayoclinic.org/diseases-conditions/burning-mouth-syndrome/basics/symptoms/con-20029596.

Burning mouth syndrome Tests and diagnosis. (2015). Retrieved on January 22, 2015, from http://www.mayoclinic.org/diseases-conditions/burning-mouth-syndrome/basics/tests-diagnosis/con-20029596.

Burning mouth syndrome. DermNet NZ. (2015). Retrieved on January 22, 2015, from http://www.dermnetnz.org/site-age-specific/burning-mouth.html.

Burning mouth syndrome. (2015). Retrieved on January 22, 2015, from http://en.wikipedia.org/wiki/Burning_mouth_syndrome.

How can I relieve the burning in my mouth? – The Chart. (2015). Retrieved on January 22, 2015, from http://thechart.blogs.cnn.com/2010/08/19/how-can-i-relieve-the-burning-in-my-mouth/comment-page-1/.

Natural Cures for Burning Mouth Syndrome. (2015). Retrieved on January 22, 2015, from http://www.earthclinic.com/cures/burning-mouth-syndrome.html.

Tell me about › Sundry › Burning mouth syndrome | The British .... (2015). Retrieved on January 22, 2015, from https://www.dentalhealth.org/tell-me-about/topic/sundry/burning-mouth-syndrome.

Tongue Burn: Causes, Risk Factors & Symptoms. (2015). Retrieved on January 22, 2015, from http://www.healthline.com/health/tongue-burn.

What's causing the burning sensation in my mouth?. (2015). Retrieved on January 22, 2015, from http://www.askdoctork.com/whats-causing-the-burning-sensation-in-my-mouth-201304184710.

Life Enhancement Products. (2015). *Lipoic Acid Helps Quench the Fire of Burning Mouth Syndrome.* Retrieved on January 22, 2015, from http://www.life-enhancement.com/magazine/article/726-lipoic-acid-helps-quench-the-fire-of-burning-mouth-syndrome.

Nick Senzee. (2015). *Burning Mouth Syndrome.* Retrieved on January 22, 2015, from http://www.aaom.com/index.php?option=com_content&view=article&id=81:burning-mouth-syndrome&catid=22:patient-condition-information&Itemid=120.

Penza P , et al.. (2015). . Retrieved on January 22, 2015, from http://www.ncbi.nlm.nih.gov/pubmed/20551728.

Suarez P and Clark GT. (2015). *Burning mouth syndrome: an update on diagnosis and treatment ....* Retrieved on January 22, 2015, from http://www.ncbi.nlm.nih.gov/pubmed/16967671.

CHAPTER 7

PATHOPHYSIOLOGY

Understanding Pathophysiology

Pathophysiology is used to describe the changes that occur in the body in response to injury or disease. The term pathophysiology is actually the combination of two words, **pathology** and **physiology**.

The human body constantly works to maintain homeostasis, meaning an internal stability between all the interdependent functions and processes that combine to keep human biological processes functioning in a normal, healthy manner. When activities of the body can not maintain homeostasis, disease ensues. Pathology is the scientific study of disease and pathologists are medical professionals who specialize in diagnosing disease. More specifically, the field of pathology is concerned with identifying the nature and physical origin and course of disease. Within the framework of pathology, the related concept **pathogenesis** focuses exclusively on the origin of disease.

On the other hand, physiology is the branch of biology that studies the physical and chemical functions and processes in living organisms. In this regard, human physiologists research the growth and development requirements of the human body, the absorption and use of nutrients to to fuel energy, and the healthy functioning of organs, tissues, and other anatomical structures. For our purposes, the most important distinction between the fields of human pathology and physiology is the former is concerned with the study of the body in a diseased state and the latter is concerned with the body in a healthy state. Therefore, pathophysiology can be thought of as the study of how disease alters the normal biological and chemical processes in a healthy human body.

Burning Mouth Syndrome Journal Articles

Al Quran, F. A. M. (2004). Psychological profile in burning mouth syndrome. *Oral Surgery, Oral Medicine, Oral Pathology, Oral Radiology, and Endodontics, 97*(3), 339–344. http://doi.org/10.1016/j.tripleo.2003.09.017

Balasubramaniam, R., Klasser, G. D., & Delcanho, R. (2009). Separating oral burning from burning mouth syndrome: Unravelling a diagnostic enigma. *Australian Dental Journal.* http://doi.org/10.1111/j.1834-7819.2009.01153.x

Barker, K. E., & Savage, N. W. (2005). Burning mouth syndrome: An update on recent findings. *Australian Dental Journal.* http://doi.org/10.1111/j.1834-7819.2005.tb00363.x

Boy-Metin, Z., Kayhan, K. B., & Unür, M. (2008). Burning mouth syndrome. *Kulak Burun Boğaz Ihtisas Dergisi : KBB = Journal of Ear, Nose, and Throat, 18*(3), 188–96. Retrieved from http://www.ncbi.nlm.nih.gov/pubmed/19388467

Brufau-Redondo, C., Martín-Brufau, R., Corbalán-Velez, R., & De Concepción-Salesa, a. (2002). Burning mouth syndrome. *British Dental Journal, 45*(6), 237–241. http://doi.org/10.1111/j.1526-4637.2010.01035.x

Cerchiari, D. P., de Moricz, R. D., Sanjar, F. A., Rapoport, P. B., Moretti, G., & Guerra, M. M. (2006). Burning mouth syndrome: etiology. *Brazilian Journal of Otorhinolaryngology, 72*(3), 419–23. http://doi.org/S0034-72992006000300021 [pii]

Charleston, L. th. (2013). Burning mouth syndrome: a review of recent literature. *Curr Pain Headache Rep, 17*(6), 336. http://doi.org/10.1007/s11916-013-0336-9

Cibirka, R. M., Nelson, S. K., & Lefebvre, C. A. (1999). A review of burning mouth syndrome. *The Journal of Prosthetic Dentistry, 78*(1), 29–35.

Coon, E. A., & Laughlin, R. S. (2012). Burning mouth syndrome in Parkinson's disease: Dopamine as cure or cause? *Journal of Headache and Pain, 13*(3), 255–257. http://doi.org/10.1007/s10194-012-0421-1

Crow, H. C., & Gonzalez, Y. (2012). Burning Mouth Syndrome. *Oral and Maxillofacial Surgery Clinics of North America, 65*(5), 343–347. http://doi.org/10.4248/IJOS10008

Crow, H. C., & Gonzalez, Y. (2013). Burning Mouth Syndrome. *Oral and*

Maxillofacial Surgery Clinics of North America.
http://doi.org/10.1016/j.coms.2012.11.001

Ducasse, D., Courtet, P., & Olie, E. (2013). Burning mouth syndrome:
current clinical, physiopathologic, and therapeutic data. *Regional Anesthesia
and Pain Medicine, 38*(5), 380–90.
http://doi.org/10.1097/AAP.0b013e3182a1f0db

Fedele, S., Fricchione, G., Porter, & Mignogna, M. (2007a). Stomatodynia or
burning mouth syndrome. *Acta Dermatovenerologica Croatica ADC
Hrvatsko Dermatolosko Drustvo, 100*(4), 231–235. Retrieved from
http://discovery.ucl.ac.uk/148057/

Fedele, S., Fricchione, G., Porter, S. R., & Mignogna, M. D. (2007b).
Stomatodynia or burning mouth syndrome. *Acta Dermatovenerologica
Croatica ADC Hrvatsko Dermatolosko Drustvo, 11*(4), 231–235. Retrieved
from http://discovery.ucl.ac.uk/148057/

Friedman, D. I. (2010). Topirimate-induced burning mouth syndrome.
Headache, 50(8), 1383–1385. http://doi.org/10.1111/j.1526-
4610.2010.01720.x

Grushka, M., Epstein, J. B., & Gorsky, M. (2002). Burning mouth syndrome.
American Family Physician, 65(4). http://doi.org/10.3748/wjg.v19.i5.665

Gurvits, G. E., & Tan, A. (2013a). Burning mouth syndrome. *World Journal
of Gastroenterology.* http://doi.org/10.3748/wjg.v19.i5.665

Gurvits, G. E., & Tan, A. (2013b). Burning mouth syndrome. *World Journal
of Gastroenterology : WJG, 19*(5), 665–72.
http://doi.org/10.3748/wjg.v19.i5.665

Hagelberg, N., Forssell, H., Rinne, J. O., Scheinin, H., Taiminen, T., Aalto,
S., … Jääskeläinen, S. (2003). Striatal dopamine D1 and D2 receptors in
burning mouth syndrome. *Pain, 101*(1-2), 149–154.
http://doi.org/10.1016/S0304-3959(02)00323-8

Huang, W., Rothe, M. J., & Grant-Kels, J. M. (1996). The burning mouth
syndrome. *Journal of the American Academy of Dermatology, 34*(1), 91–98.
http://doi.org/10.1016/S0190-9622(96)90840-3

Jääskeläinen, S. K. (2012). Pathophysiology of primary burning mouth
syndrome. *Clinical Neurophysiology.*
http://doi.org/10.1016/j.clinph.2011.07.054

Klasser, G. D., Epstein, J. B., & Villines, D. (2011). Management of burning mouth syndrome. *Journal (Canadian Dental Association)*, *77*, b151. Retrieved from http://www.ncbi.nlm.nih.gov/pubmed/22260804

Klasser, G. D., Fischer, D. J., & Epstein, J. B. (2008). Burning Mouth Syndrome: Recognition, Understanding, and Management. *Oral and Maxillofacial Surgery Clinics of North America*. http://doi.org/10.1016/j.coms.2007.12.012

Lamey, P. J., & Lamb, A. B. (1994). Lip component of burning mouth syndrome. *Oral Surgery, Oral Medicine, and Oral Pathology*, *78*(5), 590–593. http://doi.org/10.1016/0030-4220(94)90169-4

Lauria, G., Majorana, A., Borgna, M., Lombardi, R., Penza, P., Padovani, A., & Sapelli, P. (2005). Trigeminal small-fiber sensory neuropathy causes burning mouth syndrome. *Pain*, *115*(3), 332–337. http://doi.org/10.1016/j.pain.2005.03.028

López-Jornet, P., Camacho-Alonso, F., & Andujar-Mateos, P. (2011). A prospective, randomized study on the efficacy of tongue protector in patients with burning mouth syndrome. *Oral Diseases*, *17*(3), 277–282. http://doi.org/10.1111/j.1601-0825.2010.01737.x

López-Jornet, P., Camacho-Alonso, F., Andujar-Mateos, P., Sánchez-Siles, M., & Gómez-Garcia, F. (2010). Burning mouth syndrome: an update. *Medicina Oral, Patología Oral Y Cirugía Bucal*, *15*(4), e562–8. Retrieved from http://www.ncbi.nlm.nih.gov/pubmed/23772971

Marino, R., Capaccio, P., Pignataro, L., & Spadari, F. (2009). Burning mouth syndrome: The role of contact hypersensitivity. *Oral Diseases*, *15*(4), 255–258. http://doi.org/10.1111/j.1601-0825.2009.01515.x

Marino, R., Torretta, S., Capaccio, P., Pignataro, L., & Spadari, F. (2010). Different therapeutic strategies for burning mouth syndrome: preliminary data. *Journal of Oral Pathology & Medicine : Official Publication of the International Association of Oral Pathologists and the American Academy of Oral Pathology*, *39*(8), 611–616. http://doi.org/10.1111/j.1600-0714.2010.00922.x

Mignogna, M. D., Adamo, D., Schiavone, V., Ravel, M. G., & Fortuna, G. (2011). Burning Mouth Syndrome Responsive to Duloxetine: A Case Report. *Pain Medicine*, *12*(3), 466–469. http://doi.org/10.1111/j.1526-4637.2010.01035.x

Minor, J. S., & Epstein, J. B. (2011a). Burning mouth syndrome and secondary oral burning. *Otolaryngologic Clinics of North America.* http://doi.org/10.1016/j.otc.2010.09.008

Minor, J. S., & Epstein, J. B. (2011b). Burning mouth syndrome and secondary oral burning. *Otolaryngol Clin N Am, 44*(1), 205–19, vii. http://doi.org/10.1016/j.otc.2010.09.008

Mock, D., & Chugh, D. (2010). Burning mouth syndrome. *Int.J.Oral Sci., 2*(1), 1–4.

Mock, D., & Chugh, D. (2010). Burning mouth syndrome. *International Journal of Oral Science, 2*(1), 1–4. http://doi.org/10.4248/IJOS10008

Muzyka, B. C., & De Rossi, S. S. (1999). A review of burning mouth syndrome. *Cutis; Cutaneous Medicine for the Practitioner, 64*(1), 29–35.

Ni Riordain, R., Moloney, E., Osullivan, K., & McCreary, C. (2010). Burning mouth syndrome and oral health-related quality of life: Is there a change over time? *Oral Diseases, 16*(7), 643–647. http://doi.org/10.1111/j.1601-0825.2010.01666.x

Patton, L. L., Siegel, M. A., Benoliel, R., & De Laat, A. (2007). Management of burning mouth syndrome: systematic review and management recommendations. *Oral Surgery, Oral Medicine, Oral Pathology, Oral Radiology, and Endodontics, 103 Suppl,* S39.e1–e13. http://doi.org/10.1016/j.tripleo.2006.11.009

Rhodus, N. L., Carlson, C. R., & Miller, C. S. (2003). Burning mouth (syndrome) disorder. *Quintessence International (Berlin, Germany : 1985), 34*(8), 587–593.

Savage, N. W., Boras, V. V, & Barker, K. (2006). Burning mouth syndrome: clinical presentation, diagnosis and treatment. *The Australasian Journal of Dermatology, 47*(2), 77–81; quiz 82–83. http://doi.org/10.1111/j.1440-0960.2006.00236.x

Spanemberg, J. C., Cherubini, K., De Figueiredo, M. A. Z., Yurgel, L. S., & Salum, F. G. (2012). Aetiology and therapeutics of burning mouth syndrome: An update. *Gerodontology.* http://doi.org/10.1111/j.1741-2358.2010.00384.x

Speciali, J. G., & Stuginski-Barbosa, J. (2008). Burning mouth syndrome. *Current Pain and Headache Reports.* http://doi.org/10.1007/s11916-008-0047-9

Speciali, J. G., & Stuginski-Barbosa, J. (2008). Burning mouth syndrome. *Curr Pain Headache Rep., 12*(4), 279–284.

Stuginski-Barbosa, J., Rodrigues, G. G. R., Bigal, M. E., & Speciali, J. G. (2008). Burning mouth syndrome responsive to pramipexol. *Journal of Headache and Pain, 9*(1), 43–45. http://doi.org/10.1007/s10194-008-0003-4

Suda, S., Takagai, S., Inoshima-Takahashi, K., Sugihara, G., Mori, N., & Takei, N. (2008). Electroconvulsive therapy for burning mouth syndrome. *Acta Psychiatrica Scandinavica, 118*(6), 503–504. http://doi.org/10.1111/j.1600-0447.2008.01261.x

Sun, A., Wu, K.-M., Wang, Y.-P., Lin, H.-P., Chen, H.-M., & Chiang, C.-P. (2013). Burning mouth syndrome: a review and update. *Journal of Oral Pathology & Medicine : Official Publication of the International Association of Oral Pathologists and the American Academy of Oral Pathology, 42*, 649–55. http://doi.org/10.1111/jop.12101

Thoppay, J. R., De Rossi, S. S., & Ciarrocca, K. N. (2013). Burning mouth syndrome. *Dental Clinics of North America.* http://doi.org/10.1016/j.cden.2013.04.010

Torgerson, R. R. (2010). Burning mouth syndrome. *Dermatologic Therapy.* http://doi.org/10.1111/j.1529-8019.2010.01325.x

Torgerson, R. R. (2010). Burning mouth syndrome. *Dermatol Ther, 23*(3), 291–298. http://doi.org/DTH1325 [pii]\r10.1111/j.1529-8019.2010.01325.x [doi]

Wandeur, T., De Moura, S. A. B., De Medeiros, A. M. C., MacHado, M. A. N., De Azevedo Alanis, L. R., Grégio, A. M. T., … De Lima, A. A. S. (2011). Exfoliative cytology of the oral mucosa in burning mouth syndrome: A cytomorphological and cytomorphometric analysis. *Gerodontology, 28*(1), 44–48. http://doi.org/10.1111/j.1741-2358.2009.00319.x

Zur, E. (2012). Burning mouth syndrome: a discussion of a complex pathology. *International Journal of Pharmaceutical Compounding, 16*(3), 196–205. Retrieved from http://www.ncbi.nlm.nih.gov/pubmed/23050296\nhttp://www.scopus.com/inw eid=2-s2.0-84868250574&partnerID=tZOtx3y1

Burning Mouth Syndrome Internet Articles and Research

BURNING MOUTH SYNDROME: A REVIEW AND UPDATE – JPDA.

(2015). Retrieved on January 22, 2015, from
http://www.jpda.com.pk/burning-mouth-syndrome-a-review-and-update/.

Burning Mouth Syndrome. (2015). Retrieved on January 22, 2015, from
http://bjp.sagepub.com/content/5/4/12.refs.

Burning Mouth Syndrome. (2015). Retrieved on January 22, 2015, from
http://emedicine.medscape.com/article/1508869-overview.

Burning Mouth Syndrome. (2015). Retrieved on January 22, 2015, from
http://oto.sagepub.com/content/143/2_suppl/P159.1.full.

Burning Mouth Syndrome. (2015). Retrieved on January 22, 2015, from
http://www.aafp.org/afp/2002/0215/p615.html.

Burning Mouth Syndrome. (2015). Retrieved on January 22, 2015, from
http://www.practicalpainmanagement.com/pain/maxillofacial/burning-mouth-
syndrome.

Burning mouth syndrome (stomatodynia) | QJM: An International .... (2015).
Retrieved on January 22, 2015, from
http://qjmed.oxfordjournals.org/content/100/8/527.

Burning mouth syndrome. DermNet NZ. (2015). Retrieved on January 22,
2015, from http://www.dermnetnz.org/site-age-specific/burning-mouth.html.

Burning mouth syndrome: A review on its diagnostic and therapeutic ....
(2015). Retrieved on January 22, 2015, from
http://www.jpbsonline.org/article.asp?issn=0975-
7406;year=2014;volume=6;issue=5;spage=21;epage=25;aulast=Aravindhan.

Clinics. (2015). Retrieved on January 22, 2015, from
http://www.scielo.br/scielo.php?pid=S1807-
59322011000300026&script=sci_arttext.

Temporomandibular Disorders in Burning Mouth Syndrome Patients ....
(2015). Retrieved on January 22, 2015, from
http://www.medsci.org/v10p1784.htm.

Update on Burning Mouth Syndrome: Overview and Patient .... (2015).
Retrieved on January 22, 2015, from
http://cro.sagepub.com/content/14/4/275.full.

Xerostomia. (2015). Retrieved on January 22, 2015, from
http://en.wikipedia.org/wiki/Xerostomia.

Jääskeläinen SK. (2015). *Pathophysiology of primary burning mouth syndrome.*. Retrieved on January 22, 2015, from http://www.ncbi.nlm.nih.gov/pubmed/22030140.

Scott Moses, MD. (2015). *Burning Mouth Syndrome.* Retrieved on January 22, 2015, from http://www.fpnotebook.com/ent/sx/BrngMthSyndrm.htm.

CHAPTER 8

TREATMENT

Once a diagnosis Burning Mouth Syndrome has been confirmed, a patient generally begins a treatment regime under the supervision of a doctor or other medical specialist. This Chapter defines the terms **treatment** and **therapy** and discusses the most common treatment protocols for Burning Mouth Syndrome.

Treatment and Therapy

The term treatment refers to any method used by a person to remedy a health problem. Treatment can also mean doing nothing at all, often termed to "wath and wait." In medicine, treatment is often referred to as **therapy** and for our purposes the terms treatment and therapy will be used synonymously, both being based on the Greek origin of the word "therapy," to mean "curing or healing."

Treatment or therapy can be applied both to a person's biological being as well to their psychological state. Additionally, treatment can be used to remedy or halt the progression of an existing health condition **(abortive therapy)**, prevent the manifestation of a condition in an otherwise healthy person **(prophylatic therapy)**, or increase the comfort or emotional well-being of a patient when an underlying condition can not be completely eliminated **(palliative therapy)**.

During the course of your research, you will discover that the administration of certain treatments, particularly drug treatments, are often qualified by the terms **indications** and **contraindications**. Indications simply describe the circumstances and conditions that should be present before a particular treatment is administered to a patient. One common indication for drug therapies is that a patient avoid alcohol or refrain from eating for a certain period of time prior to taking a medication. Conversely, a contraindication are circumstances where a treatment should not be administered. For example, some drug treatments or physical therapy activities should not be administered in persons with high blood pressure.

There are two types of contraindications, **relative contraindications** and **absolute contraindications**. Relative contraindications occur if caution should be taken when using two or more therapies simultaneously. For therapies with relative contraindications multiple treatments should only be employed if the benefits of using more than one treatment are likely to outweigh the risks. As the term suggests, absolute contraindications means two or more treatments should not be simultaneously administred under any circumstance, as the result could cause death or serious and permanent damage. Obviously, depending on how the treatment instructions are worded some indications for treatment can become contraindications with the addition of words like "not" or "don't."

Unlike indications and contraindications, **side effects** of treatment or therapy refers to any effect in addition to, or on top of, the intended effect of the treatment. The term side effect is most commonly used when referring to drug therapies and while effects can be positive, they are most commonly negative or harmful but seldom cause serious or permanent biological or psychological damage.

Finally, therapies are also referred to as either being **first-line therapies** or **second-line therapies**. Quite simply, first-line therapies refer to the first or preferred treatment options and second-line therapies are commonly employed only when the first-line therapy doesn't produce the desirable outcome or if the patient has other health concerns that make the first-line therapy ill-advised because of complications or contraindications.

Burning Mouth Syndrome Journal Articles

Al Quran, F. A. M. (2004). Psychological profile in burning mouth syndrome. *Oral Surgery, Oral Medicine, Oral Pathology, Oral Radiology, and Endodontics, 97*(3), 339–344. http://doi.org/10.1016/j.tripleo.2003.09.017

Barker, K. E., Batstone, M. D., & Savage, N. W. (2009). Comparison of treatment modalities in burning mouth syndrome. *Australian Dental Journal, 54*(4), 300–305. http://doi.org/10.1111/j.1834-7819.2009.01154.x

Barker, K. E., & Savage, N. W. (2005). Burning mouth syndrome: An update on recent findings. *Australian Dental Journal.* http://doi.org/10.1111/j.1834-7819.2005.tb00363.x

Brufau-Redondo, C., Martín-Brufau, R., Corbalán-Velez, R., & De Concepción-Salesa, a. (2002). Burning mouth syndrome. *British Dental Journal, 45*(6), 237–241. http://doi.org/10.1111/j.1526-4637.2010.01035.x

Cerchiari, D. P., de Moricz, R. D., Sanjar, F. A., Rapoport, P. B., Moretti, G., & Guerra, M. M. (2006). Burning mouth syndrome: etiology. *Brazilian Journal of Otorhinolaryngology, 72*(3), 419–23. http://doi.org/S0034-72992006000300021 [pii]

Cibirka, R. M., Nelson, S. K., & Lefebvre, C. A. (1999). A review of burning mouth syndrome. *The Journal of Prosthetic Dentistry, 78*(1), 29–35.

Coon, E. A., & Laughlin, R. S. (2012). Burning mouth syndrome in Parkinson's disease: Dopamine as cure or cause? *Journal of Headache and Pain, 13*(3), 255–257. http://doi.org/10.1007/s10194-012-0421-1

Crow, H. C., & Gonzalez, Y. (2012). Burning Mouth Syndrome. *Oral and Maxillofacial Surgery Clinics of North America, 65*(5), 343–347. http://doi.org/10.4248/IJOS10008

Crow, H. C., & Gonzalez, Y. (2013). Burning Mouth Syndrome. *Oral and Maxillofacial Surgery Clinics of North America.* http://doi.org/10.1016/j.coms.2012.11.001

De Moraes, M., do Amaral Bezerra, B. A., da Rocha Neto, P. C., de Oliveira Soares, A. C. A., Pinto, L. P., & de Lisboa Lopes Costa, A. (2012). Randomized trials for the treatment of burning mouth syndrome: an evidence-based review of the literature. *Journal of Oral Pathology & Medicine : Official Publication of the International Association of Oral*

Pathologists and the American Academy of Oral Pathology, 41(4), 281–7. http://doi.org/10.1111/j.1600-0714.2011.01100.x

Ducasse, D., Courtet, P., & Olie, E. (2013). Burning mouth syndrome: current clinical, physiopathologic, and therapeutic data. *Regional Anesthesia and Pain Medicine, 38*(5), 380–90. http://doi.org/10.1097/AAP.0b013e3182a1f0db

Fedele, S., Fricchione, G., Porter, & Mignogna, M. (2007a). Stomatodynia or burning mouth syndrome. *Acta Dermatovenerologica Croatica ADC Hrvatsko Dermatolosko Drustvo, 100*(4), 231–235. Retrieved from http://discovery.ucl.ac.uk/148057/

Fedele, S., Fricchione, G., Porter, S. R., & Mignogna, M. D. (2007b). Stomatodynia or burning mouth syndrome. *Acta Dermatovenerologica Croatica ADC Hrvatsko Dermatolosko Drustvo, 11*(4), 231–235. Retrieved from http://discovery.ucl.ac.uk/148057/

Friedman, D. I. (2010). Topirimate-induced burning mouth syndrome. *Headache, 50*(8), 1383–1385. http://doi.org/10.1111/j.1526-4610.2010.01720.x

Grushka, M., Epstein, J. B., & Gorsky, M. (2002a). Burning mouth syndrome. *American Family Physician, 65*(4). http://doi.org/10.3748/wjg.v19.i5.665

Grushka, M., Epstein, J. B., & Gorsky, M. (2002). Burning mouth syndrome. *Am Fam Physician, 65*(4), 615–620. Retrieved from http://www.ncbi.nlm.nih.gov/entrez/query.fcgi?cmd=Retrieve&db=PubMed&dopt=Citation&list_uids=11871678

Grushka, M., Epstein, J., & Gorsky, M. (2002b). Burning mouth syndrome. *American Family Physician, 65*(4), 615–620. Retrieved from http://www.ncbi.nlm.nih.gov/pubmed/11871678

Gurvits, G. E., & Tan, A. (2013). Burning mouth syndrome. *World Journal of Gastroenterology : WJG, 19*(5), 665–72. http://doi.org/10.3748/wjg.v19.i5.665

Jääskeläinen, S. K. (2012). Pathophysiology of primary burning mouth syndrome. *Clinical Neurophysiology.* http://doi.org/10.1016/j.clinph.2011.07.054

Klasser, G. D., Fischer, D. J., & Epstein, J. B. (2008). Burning Mouth

Syndrome: Recognition, Understanding, and Management. *Oral and Maxillofacial Surgery Clinics of North America.* http://doi.org/10.1016/j.coms.2007.12.012

Lamey, P. J., & Lamb, A. B. (1994). Lip component of burning mouth syndrome. *Oral Surgery, Oral Medicine, and Oral Pathology, 78*(5), 590–593. http://doi.org/10.1016/0030-4220(94)90169-4

López-Jornet, P., Camacho-Alonso, F., & Andujar-Mateos, P. (2011). A prospective, randomized study on the efficacy of tongue protector in patients with burning mouth syndrome. *Oral Diseases, 17*(3), 277–282. http://doi.org/10.1111/j.1601-0825.2010.01737.x

López-Jornet, P., Camacho-Alonso, F., Andujar-Mateos, P., Sánchez-Siles, M., & Gómez-Garcia, F. (2010). Burning mouth syndrome: an update. *Medicina Oral, Patología Oral Y Cirugía Bucal, 15*(4), e562–8. Retrieved from http://www.ncbi.nlm.nih.gov/pubmed/23772971

López-Jornet, P., Camacho-Alonso, F., & Leon-Espinosa, S. (2009). Efficacy of alpha lipoic acid in burning mouth syndrome: A randomized, placebo-treatment study. *Journal of Oral Rehabilitation, 36*(1), 52–57. http://doi.org/10.1111/j.1365-2842.2008.01914.x

Maltsman-Tseikhin, A., Moricca, P., & Niv, D. (2007). Burning mouth syndrome: will better understanding yield better management? *Pain Practice : The Official Journal of World Institute of Pain, 7*(2), 151–162. http://doi.org/10.1111/j.1533-2500.2007.00124.x

Marino, R., Capaccio, P., Pignataro, L., & Spadari, F. (2009). Burning mouth syndrome: The role of contact hypersensitivity. *Oral Diseases, 15*(4), 255–258. http://doi.org/10.1111/j.1601-0825.2009.01515.x

McGirr, A., Davis, L., & Vila-Rodriguez, F. (2014). Idiopathic burning mouth syndrome: A common treatment-refractory somatoform condition responsive to ECT. *Psychiatry Research, 216*(1), 158–159. http://doi.org/10.1016/j.psychres.2014.01.048

Mínguez Serra, M. P., Salort Llorca, C., & Silvestre Donat, F. J. (2007). Pharmacological treatment of burning mouth syndrome: A review and update. *Medicina Oral, Patología Oral Y Cirugía Bucal.*

Minor, J. S., & Epstein, J. B. (2011a). Burning mouth syndrome and secondary oral burning. *Otolaryngologic Clinics of North America.* http://doi.org/10.1016/j.otc.2010.09.008

Minor, J. S., & Epstein, J. B. (2011b). Burning mouth syndrome and secondary oral burning. *Otolaryngol Clin N Am, 44*(1), 205–19, vii. http://doi.org/10.1016/j.otc.2010.09.008

Mock, D., & Chugh, D. (2010). Burning mouth syndrome. *International Journal of Oral Science, 2*(1), 1–4. http://doi.org/10.4248/IJOS10008

Muzyka, B. C., & De Rossi, S. S. (1999). A review of burning mouth syndrome. *Cutis; Cutaneous Medicine for the Practitioner, 64*(1), 29–35.

Pinto, A., Stoopler, E. T., DeRossi, S. S., Sollecito, T. P., & Popovic, R. (2002). Burning mouth syndrome: a guide for the general practitioner. *General Dentistry, 51*(5), 458–61; quiz 462. Retrieved from http://www.ncbi.nlm.nih.gov/pubmed/15055637

Rhodus, N. L., Carlson, C. R., & Miller, C. S. (2003). Burning mouth (syndrome) disorder. *Quintessence International (Berlin, Germany : 1985), 34*(8), 587–593.

Rodriguez-Cerdeira. (2012). Treatment of Burning Mouth Syndrome With Amisulpride. *Journal of Clinical Medicine Research.* http://doi.org/10.4021/jocmr972w

Savage, N. W., Boras, V. V, & Barker, K. (2006). Burning mouth syndrome: clinical presentation, diagnosis and treatment. *The Australasian Journal of Dermatology, 47*(2), 77–81; quiz 82–83. http://doi.org/10.1111/j.1440-0960.2006.00236.x

Silvestre, F. J., Silvestre-Rangil, J., Tamarit-Santafé, C., & Bautista, D. (2012). Application of a capsaicin rinse in the treatment of burning mouth syndrome. *Medicina Oral, Patologia Oral Y Cirugia Bucal, 17*(1). http://doi.org/10.4317/medoral.17219

Spanemberg, J. C., Cherubini, K., De Figueiredo, M. A. Z., Yurgel, L. S., & Salum, F. G. (2012). Aetiology and therapeutics of burning mouth syndrome: An update. *Gerodontology.* http://doi.org/10.1111/j.1741-2358.2010.00384.x

Speciali, J. G., & Stuginski-Barbosa, J. (2008). Burning mouth syndrome. *Current Pain and Headache Reports.* http://doi.org/10.1007/s11916-008-0047-9

Speciali, J. G., & Stuginski-Barbosa, J. (2008). Burning mouth syndrome. *Curr Pain Headache Rep., 12*(4), 279–284.

Stuginski-Barbosa, J., Rodrigues, G. G. R., Bigal, M. E., & Speciali, J. G.

(2008). Burning mouth syndrome responsive to pramipexol. *Journal of Headache and Pain*, 9(1), 43–45. http://doi.org/10.1007/s10194-008-0003-4

Suda, S., Takagai, S., Inoshima-Takahashi, K., Sugihara, G., Mori, N., & Takei, N. (2008). Electroconvulsive therapy for burning mouth syndrome. *Acta Psychiatrica Scandinavica*, *118*(6), 503–504. http://doi.org/10.1111/j.1600-0447.2008.01261.x

Sun, A., Wu, K.-M., Wang, Y.-P., Lin, H.-P., Chen, H.-M., & Chiang, C.-P. (2013). Burning mouth syndrome: a review and update. *Journal of Oral Pathology & Medicine : Official Publication of the International Association of Oral Pathologists and the American Academy of Oral Pathology*, *42*, 649–55. http://doi.org/10.1111/jop.12101

Thoppay, J. R., De Rossi, S. S., & Ciarrocca, K. N. (2013). Burning mouth syndrome. *Dental Clinics of North America*. http://doi.org/10.1016/j.cden.2013.04.010

Torgerson, R. R. (2010). Burning mouth syndrome. *Dermatologic Therapy*. http://doi.org/10.1111/j.1529-8019.2010.01325.x

Yan, Z., Ding, N., & Hua, H. (2012). A systematic review of acupuncture or acupoint injection for management of burning mouth syndrome. *Quintessence International (Berlin, Germany : 1985)*. Retrieved from http://www.ncbi.nlm.nih.gov/pubmed/23034422

Yang, H.-W., & Huang, Y.-F. (2011). Treatment of burning mouth syndrome with a low-level energy diode laser. *Photomedicine and Laser Surgery*, *29*(2), 123–125. http://doi.org/10.1089/pho.2010.2787

Zakrzewska, J. M., Forssell, H., & Glenny, A. M. (2005). Interventions for the treatment of burning mouth syndrome. *The Cochrane Database of Systematic Reviews*, (1), CD002779. http://doi.org/10.1002/14651858.CD002779.pub2

Zakrzewska, J. M., Forssell, H., & Glenny, A.-M. (2003). Interventions for the treatment of burning mouth syndrome: a systematic review. *Journal of Orofacial Pain*, *17*(4), 293–300.

Zur, E. (2012). Burning mouth syndrome: a discussion of a complex pathology. *International Journal of Pharmaceutical Compounding*, *16*(3), 196–205. Retrieved from http://www.ncbi.nlm.nih.gov/pubmed/23050296\nhttp://www.scopus.com/inw eid=2-s2.0-84868250574&partnerID=tZOtx3y1

Burning Mouth Syndrome Internet Articles and Research

Burning Mouth Syndrome (Glossopyrosis) Medication | Drugs.com. (2015). Retrieved on January 22, 2015, from http://www.drugs.com/condition/burning-mouth-syndrome.html.

Burning Mouth Syndrome | Overview. (2015). Retrieved on January 22, 2015, from http://familydoctor.org/familydoctor/en/diseases-conditions/burning-mouth-syndrome.html.

Burning Mouth Syndrome: Causes and Treatment Options – 1. (2015). Retrieved on January 22, 2015, from http://www.1800dentist.com/burning-mouth-syndrome/.

Burning Mouth Syndrome: Learn About Symptoms. (2015). Retrieved on January 22, 2015, from http://www.medicinenet.com/burning_mouth_syndrome/article.htm.

Burning Mouth Syndrome. (2015). Retrieved on January 22, 2015, from http://emedicine.medscape.com/article/1508869-overview.

Burning Mouth Syndrome. (2015). Retrieved on January 22, 2015, from http://www.aafp.org/afp/2002/0215/p615.html.

Burning Mouth Syndrome. (2015). Retrieved on January 22, 2015, from http://www.colgateprofessional.com/patient-education/articles/burning-mouth-syndrome.

Burning Mouth Syndrome. (2015). Retrieved on January 22, 2015, from http://www.nidcr.nih.gov/oralhealth/Topics/Burning/BurningMouthSyndrome

Burning Mouth Syndrome. (2015). Retrieved on January 22, 2015, from http://www.sharecare.com/health/burning-mouth-syndrome.

Burning Mouth Syndrome. (2015). Retrieved on January 22, 2015, from http://www.webmd.com/oral-health/burning-mouth-syndrome.

Burning Mouth Syndrome. (2015). Retrieved on January 22, 2015, from http://www.yourdentistryguide.com/burning-mouth/.

Burning Mouth. (2015). Retrieved on January 22, 2015, from http://my.clevelandclinic.org/health/diseases_conditions/hic_burning_mouth.

Burning Tongue Syndrome | 34. (2015). Retrieved on January 22, 2015, from http://www.34-menopause-symptoms.com/burning-tongue/articles/burning-tongue-syndrome.htm.

Burning Tongue | 34. (2015). Retrieved on January 22, 2015, from http://www.34-menopause-symptoms.com/burning-tongue.htm.

Burning mouth syndrome Appointments. (2015). Retrieved on January 22, 2015, from http://www.mayoclinic.org/diseases-conditions/burning-mouth-syndrome/care-at-mayo-clinic/appointments/con-20029596.

Burning mouth syndrome. DermNet NZ. (2015). Retrieved on January 22, 2015, from http://www.dermnetnz.org/site-age-specific/burning-mouth.html.

Burning mouth syndrome. (2015). Retrieved on January 22, 2015, from http://en.wikipedia.org/wiki/Burning_mouth_syndrome.

Burning mouth syndrome. (2015). Retrieved on January 22, 2015, from http://www.aaomp.org/public/burning-mouth.php.

How can I relieve the burning in my mouth? – The Chart. (2015). Retrieved on January 22, 2015, from http://thechart.blogs.cnn.com/2010/08/19/how-can-i-relieve-the-burning-in-my-mouth/comment-page-1/.

Natural Cures for Burning Mouth Syndrome. (2015). Retrieved on January 22, 2015, from http://www.earthclinic.com/cures/burning-mouth-syndrome.html.

Patient Comments: Burning Mouth Syndrome. (2015). Retrieved on January 22, 2015, from http://www.medicinenet.com/burning_mouth_syndrome/patient-comments-2967.htm.

Tongue Burn: Causes, Risk Factors & Symptoms. (2015). Retrieved on January 22, 2015, from http://www.healthline.com/health/tongue-burn.

ABC News. (2015). *The Mysterious, Agonizing Pain of Burning Mouth Syndrome.* Retrieved on January 22, 2015, from http://abcnews.go.com/Health/PainManagement/story?id=4274230.

Life Enhancement Products. (2015). *Lipoic Acid Helps Quench the Fire of Burning Mouth Syndrome.* Retrieved on January 22, 2015, from http://www.life-enhancement.com/magazine/article/726-lipoic-acid-helps-quench-the-fire-of-burning-mouth-syndrome.

Nick Senzee. (2015). *Burning Mouth Syndrome.* Retrieved on January 22, 2015, from http://www.aaom.com/index.php?option=com_content&view=article&id=81:burning-mouth-syndrome&catid=22:patient-condition-information&Itemid=120.

Suarez P and Clark GT. (2015). *Burning mouth syndrome: an update on diagnosis and treatment* .... Retrieved on January 22, 2015, from http://www.ncbi.nlm.nih.gov/pubmed/16967671.

CHAPTER 9

PROGNOSIS

Defining Prognosis

A prognosis is a forecast as to the probable outcome or status of a disease or health condition at a defined point in time in the future. It is most often used to refer to the estimated chance of survival or recovery, though it can also refer to the chances of complications, the time to recovery, or other probable or possible outcomes.

While a prognosis is most frequently phrased in percentage terms, "the patient with Disease X has a 85% chance of survival," it is ultimately only an opinion made by a doctor, even though the doctor refers to medical research of past outcomes for similarly situated patients to form his opinion. In Biomedical Research, making generalizations about patient prognoses is steeped heavily not only in the biological sciences but in mathematical science and statistics as well, in a field known as "Survival Analysis."

Survival analysis can be defined as a group of statistical methods used to analyze and evaluate data to determine the time to the occurrence of an event. When applied to medicine, the event occurrence, or outcome variable, can be death, the onset a disease, the time necessary for a therapy to be effective, the progression of symptoms, and so forth. Typically, this analytic procedure is performed as part of a larger medical study of a representative sample of patients. In survival analysis data collection is quite straightforward and simply involves observing a patient over time and recording relevant information about the patient at specified intervals.

Once all data is collected, a form of regression analysis (most often the Cox Proportional Hazards Regression model) can be performed. Regression analysis evaluates the change in one or more variables (dependent variables) based on the presence of a second variable or set of variables (independent variables). In survival analysis the independent variable is commonly the presence of a disease or health condition and dependent variables almost always include both an event status (whether an event did or did not occur) and the time to occurrence of the event. A simple example is predicting the time to death for individuals with inoperable lung cancer. In this case the independent variable is the presence of lung cancer and the dependent variables could be death (the event occurrence) and the number of days or years (time) to the death event. Based on the amount of data collected, survival analysis can also get much more specific by making separate determinations based on patient gender, age, the introduction of specific therapies, etc. To account for unique study cases, such as patients who don't die during the duration of the study period or patients who leave a study before death, a special estimator known as the Kaplan-Meier estimator is used to allow researchers to include these cases in study data but still make certain estimates are accurate.

Therefore, a prognosis simply puts in percentage terms the most likely outcome for a patient based on specific factors or variables but does not necessarily mean the event occurrence will occur in every case or, when it does, in the exact time period identified in the prognosis. Remember the research to determine a prognosis is based on hundreds and even thousands of unique cases for unique individuals and is generally only a statement of the most common outcome for the majority, or even plurality, of participants in the study. Put simply then, not all participants likely experienced the same outcome. For this reason, doctors are often hesitant to provide patients with a concrete prognosis since for some diseases and/or the unique characteristics of an individual patient actual outcomes can vary substantially from a common prognosis. This is especially true when research demonstrates multiple potential outcomes are possible. This concept is most clearly illustrated when individuals or the popular media declare a positive outcome of a disease to be a "medical miracle" even though a doctor may deem the same outcome well within the range of medical possibilities. Conversely, absent medical error, negative outcomes when compared to the prognosis given have also become the basis for countless unsuccessful lawsuits claiming medical malpractice.

Burning Mouth Syndrome Journal Articles

Al Quran, F. A. M. (2004). Psychological profile in burning mouth syndrome. *Oral Surgery, Oral Medicine, Oral Pathology, Oral Radiology, and Endodontics, 97*(3), 339–344. http://doi.org/10.1016/j.tripleo.2003.09.017

Balasubramaniam, R., Klasser, G. D., & Delcanho, R. (2009). Separating oral burning from burning mouth syndrome: Unravelling a diagnostic enigma. *Australian Dental Journal.* http://doi.org/10.1111/j.1834-7819.2009.01153.x

Barker, K. E., & Savage, N. W. (2005). Burning mouth syndrome: An update on recent findings. *Australian Dental Journal.* http://doi.org/10.1111/j.1834-7819.2005.tb00363.x

Boy-Metin, Z., Kayhan, K. B., & Unür, M. (2008). Burning mouth syndrome. *Kulak Burun Boğaz Ihtisas Dergisi : KBB = Journal of Ear, Nose, and Throat, 18*(3), 188–96. Retrieved from http://www.ncbi.nlm.nih.gov/pubmed/19388467

Brufau-Redondo, C., Martín-Brufau, R., Corbalán-Velez, R., & De Concepción-Salesa, a. (2002). Burning mouth syndrome. *British Dental Journal, 45*(6), 237–241. http://doi.org/10.1111/j.1526-4637.2010.01035.x

Brufau-Redondo, C., Martin-Brufau, R., Corbalan-Velez, R., & de Concepcion-Salesa, A. (2008). {[}Burning mouth syndrome{]}. *Actas Dermosifiliogr, 99*(6), 431–440.

Cerchiari, D. P., de Moricz, R. D., Sanjar, F. A., Rapoport, P. B., Moretti, G., & Guerra, M. M. (2006). Burning mouth syndrome: etiology. *Brazilian Journal of Otorhinolaryngology, 72*(3), 419–23. http://doi.org/S0034-72992006000300021 [pii]

Cibirka, R. M., Nelson, S. K., & Lefebvre, C. A. (1999). A review of burning mouth syndrome. *The Journal of Prosthetic Dentistry, 78*(1), 29–35.

Coon, E. A., & Laughlin, R. S. (2012). Burning mouth syndrome in Parkinson's disease: Dopamine as cure or cause? *Journal of Headache and Pain, 13*(3), 255–257. http://doi.org/10.1007/s10194-012-0421-1

Crow, H. C., & Gonzalez, Y. (2012). Burning Mouth Syndrome. *Oral and Maxillofacial Surgery Clinics of North America, 65*(5), 343–347. http://doi.org/10.4248/IJOS10008

Crow, H. C., & Gonzalez, Y. (2013). Burning Mouth Syndrome. *Oral and*

Maxillofacial Surgery Clinics of North America.
http://doi.org/10.1016/j.coms.2012.11.001

Fedele, S., Fricchione, G., Porter, & Mignogna, M. (2007a). Stomatodynia or burning mouth syndrome. *Acta Dermatovenerologica Croatica ADC Hrvatsko Dermatolosko Drustvo, 100*(4), 231–235. Retrieved from http://discovery.ucl.ac.uk/148057/

Fedele, S., Fricchione, G., Porter, S. R., & Mignogna, M. D. (2007b). Stomatodynia or burning mouth syndrome. *Acta Dermatovenerologica Croatica ADC Hrvatsko Dermatolosko Drustvo, 11*(4), 231–235. Retrieved from http://discovery.ucl.ac.uk/148057/

Forssell, H., Teerijoki-Oksa, T., Kotiranta, U., Kantola, R., Bäck, M., Vuorjoki-Ranta, T.-R., … Estlander, A.-M. (2012). Pain and pain behavior in burning mouth syndrome: a pain diary study. *Journal of Orofacial Pain, 26*(2), 117–25. Retrieved from http://www.ncbi.nlm.nih.gov/pubmed/22558611

Friedman, D. I. (2010). Topirimate-induced burning mouth syndrome. *Headache, 50*(8), 1383–1385. http://doi.org/10.1111/j.1526-4610.2010.01720.x

Gerlinger, I. (2012). [Burning sensation in oral cavity--burning mouth syndrome in everyday medical practice]. *Ideggyógyászati Szemle, 65*(9-10), 295–301. Retrieved from http://www.ncbi.nlm.nih.gov/pubmed/23126213

Grushka, M., Epstein, J. B., & Gorsky, M. (2002). Burning mouth syndrome. *American Family Physician, 65*(4). http://doi.org/10.3748/wjg.v19.i5.665

Gurvits, G. E., & Tan, A. (2013a). Burning mouth syndrome. *World Journal of Gastroenterology.* http://doi.org/10.3748/wjg.v19.i5.665

Gurvits, G. E., & Tan, A. (2013b). Burning mouth syndrome. *World Journal of Gastroenterology : WJG, 19*(5), 665–72. http://doi.org/10.3748/wjg.v19.i5.665

Hagelberg, N., Forssell, H., Rinne, J. O., Scheinin, H., Taiminen, T., Aalto, S., … Jääskeläinen, S. (2003). Striatal dopamine D1 and D2 receptors in burning mouth syndrome. *Pain, 101*(1-2), 149–154. http://doi.org/10.1016/S0304-3959(02)00323-8

Huang, W., Rothe, M. J., & Grant-Kels, J. M. (1996). The burning mouth syndrome. *Journal of the American Academy of Dermatology, 34*(1), 91–98.

http://doi.org/10.1016/S0190-9622(96)90840-3

Jääskeläinen, S. K. (2012). Pathophysiology of primary burning mouth syndrome. *Clinical Neurophysiology.* http://doi.org/10.1016/j.clinph.2011.07.054

Klasser, G. D., Epstein, J. B., & Villines, D. (2011). Management of burning mouth syndrome. *Journal (Canadian Dental Association), 77,* b151. Retrieved from http://www.ncbi.nlm.nih.gov/pubmed/22260804

Klasser, G. D., Fischer, D. J., & Epstein, J. B. (2008). Burning Mouth Syndrome: Recognition, Understanding, and Management. *Oral and Maxillofacial Surgery Clinics of North America.* http://doi.org/10.1016/j.coms.2007.12.012

Lamey, P. J., & Lamb, A. B. (1994). Lip component of burning mouth syndrome. *Oral Surgery, Oral Medicine, and Oral Pathology, 78*(5), 590–593. http://doi.org/10.1016/0030-4220(94)90169-4

Lauria, G., Majorana, A., Borgna, M., Lombardi, R., Penza, P., Padovani, A., & Sapelli, P. (2005). Trigeminal small-fiber sensory neuropathy causes burning mouth syndrome. *Pain, 115*(3), 332–337. http://doi.org/10.1016/j.pain.2005.03.028

López-Jornet, P., Camacho-Alonso, F., & Andujar-Mateos, P. (2011). A prospective, randomized study on the efficacy of tongue protector in patients with burning mouth syndrome. *Oral Diseases, 17*(3), 277–282. http://doi.org/10.1111/j.1601-0825.2010.01737.x

López-Jornet, P., Camacho-Alonso, F., Andujar-Mateos, P., Sánchez-Siles, M., & Gómez-Garcia, F. (2010). Burning mouth syndrome: an update. *Medicina Oral, Patología Oral Y Cirugía Bucal, 15*(4), e562–8. Retrieved from http://www.ncbi.nlm.nih.gov/pubmed/23772971

Marino, R., Capaccio, P., Pignataro, L., & Spadari, F. (2009). Burning mouth syndrome: The role of contact hypersensitivity. *Oral Diseases, 15*(4), 255–258. http://doi.org/10.1111/j.1601-0825.2009.01515.x

Marino, R., Torretta, S., Capaccio, P., Pignataro, L., & Spadari, F. (2010). Different therapeutic strategies for burning mouth syndrome: preliminary data. *Journal of Oral Pathology & Medicine : Official Publication of the International Association of Oral Pathologists and the American Academy of Oral Pathology, 39*(8), 611–616. http://doi.org/10.1111/j.1600-0714.2010.00922.x

Mignogna, M. D., Adamo, D., Schiavone, V., Ravel, M. G., & Fortuna, G. (2011). Burning Mouth Syndrome Responsive to Duloxetine: A Case Report. *Pain Medicine, 12*(3), 466–469. http://doi.org/10.1111/j.1526-4637.2010.01035.x

Minor, J. S., & Epstein, J. B. (2011a). Burning mouth syndrome and secondary oral burning. *Otolaryngologic Clinics of North America.* http://doi.org/10.1016/j.otc.2010.09.008

Minor, J. S., & Epstein, J. B. (2011b). Burning mouth syndrome and secondary oral burning. *Otolaryngol Clin N Am, 44*(1), 205–19, vii. http://doi.org/10.1016/j.otc.2010.09.008

Mock, D., & Chugh, D. (2010). Burning mouth syndrome. *Int.J.Oral Sci., 2*(1), 1–4.

Mock, D., & Chugh, D. (2010). Burning mouth syndrome. *International Journal of Oral Science, 2*(1), 1–4. http://doi.org/10.4248/IJOS10008

Muzyka, B. C., & De Rossi, S. S. (1999). A review of burning mouth syndrome. *Cutis; Cutaneous Medicine for the Practitioner, 64*(1), 29–35.

Nasri-Heir, C. (2012). Burning mouth syndrome. *The Alpha Omegan.*

Ni Riordain, R., Moloney, E., Osullivan, K., & McCreary, C. (2010). Burning mouth syndrome and oral health-related quality of life: Is there a change over time? *Oral Diseases, 16*(7), 643–647. http://doi.org/10.1111/j.1601-0825.2010.01666.x

Rhodus, N. L., Carlson, C. R., & Miller, C. S. (2003). Burning mouth (syndrome) disorder. *Quintessence International (Berlin, Germany : 1985), 34*(8), 587–593.

Savage, N. W., Boras, V. V, & Barker, K. (2006). Burning mouth syndrome: clinical presentation, diagnosis and treatment. *The Australasian Journal of Dermatology, 47*(2), 77–81; quiz 82–83. http://doi.org/10.1111/j.1440-0960.2006.00236.x

Spanemberg, J. C., Cherubini, K., De Figueiredo, M. A. Z., Yurgel, L. S., & Salum, F. G. (2012). Aetiology and therapeutics of burning mouth syndrome: An update. *Gerodontology.* http://doi.org/10.1111/j.1741-2358.2010.00384.x

Speciali, J. G., & Stuginski-Barbosa, J. (2008). Burning mouth syndrome. *Current Pain and Headache Reports.* http://doi.org/10.1007/s11916-008-0047-9

Stuginski-Barbosa, J., Rodrigues, G. G. R., Bigal, M. E., & Speciali, J. G. (2008). Burning mouth syndrome responsive to pramipexol. *Journal of Headache and Pain, 9*(1), 43–45. http://doi.org/10.1007/s10194-008-0003-4

Suda, S., Takagai, S., Inoshima-Takahashi, K., Sugihara, G., Mori, N., & Takei, N. (2008). Electroconvulsive therapy for burning mouth syndrome. *Acta Psychiatrica Scandinavica, 118*(6), 503–504. http://doi.org/10.1111/j.1600-0447.2008.01261.x

Sun, A., Wu, K.-M., Wang, Y.-P., Lin, H.-P., Chen, H.-M., & Chiang, C.-P. (2013). Burning mouth syndrome: a review and update. *Journal of Oral Pathology & Medicine : Official Publication of the International Association of Oral Pathologists and the American Academy of Oral Pathology, 42*, 649–55. http://doi.org/10.1111/jop.12101

Thoppay, J. R., De Rossi, S. S., & Ciarrocca, K. N. (2013). Burning mouth syndrome. *Dental Clinics of North America.* http://doi.org/10.1016/j.cden.2013.04.010

Torgerson, R. R. (2010). Burning mouth syndrome. *Dermatologic Therapy.* http://doi.org/10.1111/j.1529-8019.2010.01325.x

Wandeur, T., De Moura, S. A. B., De Medeiros, A. M. C., MacHado, M. A. N., De Azevedo Alanis, L. R., Grégio, A. M. T., … De Lima, A. A. S. (2011). Exfoliative cytology of the oral mucosa in burning mouth syndrome: A cytomorphological and cytomorphometric analysis. *Gerodontology, 28*(1), 44–48. http://doi.org/10.1111/j.1741-2358.2009.00319.x

Witt, E., & Palla, S. (2002). Mundbrennen, [Burning mouth]. *Schmerz (Berlin, Germany), 16*(5), 389–94. http://doi.org/10.1007/s00482-002-0149-y

Zur, E. (2012). Burning mouth syndrome: a discussion of a complex pathology. *International Journal of Pharmaceutical Compounding, 16*(3), 196–205. Retrieved from http://www.ncbi.nlm.nih.gov/pubmed/23050296\nhttp://www.scopus.com/inw eid=2-s2.0-84868250574&partnerID=tZOtx3y1

Burning Mouth Syndrome Internet Articles and Research

Burning Mouth Syndrome | BMS by Oral. (2015). Retrieved on January 22, 2015, from http://www.oralb.com/topics/burning-mouth-syndrome.aspx.

Burning Mouth Syndrome « University Pain Centre Maastricht. (2015). Retrieved on January 22, 2015, from http://www.pijn.com/en/patients/cause-of-pain/diagnoses-per-body-region/face-head-neck/burning-mouth-syndrome/.

Burning Mouth Syndrome: Causes and Treatment Options – 1. (2015). Retrieved on January 22, 2015, from http://www.1800dentist.com/burning-mouth-syndrome/.

Burning Mouth Syndrome: Learn About Symptoms. (2015). Retrieved on January 22, 2015, from http://www.medicinenet.com/burning_mouth_syndrome/article.htm.

Burning Mouth Syndrome. (2015). Retrieved on January 22, 2015, from http://emedicine.medscape.com/article/1508869-overview.

Burning Mouth Syndrome. (2015). Retrieved on January 22, 2015, from http://www.aafp.org/afp/2002/0215/p615.html.

Burning Mouth Syndrome. (2015). Retrieved on January 22, 2015, from http://www.nidcr.nih.gov/oralhealth/Topics/Burning/BurningMouthSyndrome

Burning mouth syndrome Appointments. (2015). Retrieved on January 22, 2015, from http://www.mayoclinic.org/diseases-conditions/burning-mouth-syndrome/care-at-mayo-clinic/appointments/con-20029596.

Burning mouth syndrome Symptoms. (2015). Retrieved on January 22, 2015, from http://www.mayoclinic.org/diseases-conditions/burning-mouth-syndrome/basics/symptoms/con-20029596.

Burning mouth syndrome as the initial sign of multiple myeloma. (2015). Retrieved on January 22, 2015, from http://www.sciencedirect.com/science/article/pii/S1741940903000062.

Burning mouth syndrome. DermNet NZ. (2015). Retrieved on January 22, 2015, from http://www.dermnetnz.org/site-age-specific/burning-mouth.html.

Burning mouth syndrome: etiology. (2015). Retrieved on January 22, 2015, from http://www.scielo.br/scielo.php?pid=s0034-72992006000300021&script=sci_arttext&tlng=en.

Burning mouth syndrome. (2015). Retrieved on January 22, 2015, from http://en.wikipedia.org/wiki/Burning_mouth_syndrome.

Burning mouth syndrome. (2015). Retrieved on January 22, 2015, from http://www.rightdiagnosis.com/b/burning_mouth_syndrome_type_3/intro.htm

Natural Cures for Burning Mouth Syndrome. (2015). Retrieved on January 22, 2015, from http://www.earthclinic.com/cures/burning-mouth-syndrome.html.

Oral Health Exam Pinpoints Burning Mouth Syndrome. (2015). Retrieved on January 22, 2015, from http://www.rdhmag.com/articles/print/volume-33/issue-10/columns/burning-mouth-syndrome.html.

Pharmacological treatment of burning mouth syndrome: A review .... (2015). Retrieved on January 22, 2015, from http://scielo.isciii.es/scielo.php?script=sci_arttext&pid=S1698-69462007000400007.

Treatments available to relieve burning mouth syndrome. (2015). Retrieved on January 22, 2015, from http://articles.sun-sentinel.com/2010-03-09/health/fl-jjps-mouth-0310-20100309_1_mouth-alpha-lipoic-acid-syndrome.

Update on Burning Mouth Syndrome: Overview and Patient .... (2015). Retrieved on January 22, 2015, from http://cro.sagepub.com/content/14/4/275.full.

We've all had burnt mouth syndrome too | Daily Mail Online. (2015). Retrieved on January 22, 2015, from http://www.dailymail.co.uk/health/article-1235316/Weve-burnt-mouth-syndrome-too.html.

Life Enhancement Products. (2015). *Lipoic Acid Helps Quench the Fire of Burning Mouth Syndrome.* Retrieved on January 22, 2015, from http://www.life-enhancement.com/magazine/article/726-lipoic-acid-helps-quench-the-fire-of-burning-mouth-syndrome.

Nasri-Heir C. (2015). *Burning mouth syndrome..* Retrieved on January 22, 2015, from http://www.ncbi.nlm.nih.gov/pubmed/23589947.

Nick Senzee. (2015). *Burning Mouth Syndrome.* Retrieved on January 22, 2015, from http://www.aaom.com/index.php?option=com_content&view=article&id=81:burning-mouth-syndrome&catid=22:patient-condition-information&Itemid=120.

CHAPTER 10

APPLIED

RESEARCH

&

RESOURCES

This final chapter provides additional resources for the reader interested in examining Burning Mouth Syndrome from a different or more in-depth perspective. Increasingly, mainstream medical researchers and doctors are recognizing how important nutrition, alternative treatments, and other so-called fringe therapies can be in preventing and treating disease. This chapter briefly provides context to these emerging therapies and identifies the best resources available for further study. Likewise, this chapter discusses additional research sources for those seeking additional information about applied research, namely information resources for those interested in the role of pharmaceuticals and biotechnology in treating disease and health conditions. Finally, this chapter provides a primer on finding and researching professional journals and other similar written publications.

Alternative Health & Complementary Medicine

More than 40% of all Americans use some form of complementary, alternative, or integrative medicine. While similar, each of these three (3) medical treatment types has a distinct meaning.

Complementary Medicine means using a non-mainstream medical approach in conjunction with conventional medicine, separating each into its own treatment. **Alternative Medicine** is when a non-mainstream medical approach is used in place or instead of a conventional approach. **Integrative Medicine** is combining a non-mainstream approach with conventional medicine to construct one unfied treatment treatment protocol.

Regardless of the exact approach, for our purposes we will describe all three together under the term Alternative Medicine. To further understand this non-mainstream medical approach it worthwhile to note that most alternative therapies have two (2) First, is the use of all natural products like herbs (botanicals), vitamins, and minerals and are collectively marketed as dietary supplements. In the past several years interest in dietary supplements has increased dramatically. The most popular supplements in recent years include fish oil and other omega 3s, ginko biloba, and echinacea. A second hallmark of most alternative medicine methods is the focus on mind and body practices. Common mind and body alternative therapies include acupuncture, massage therapy, movement therapies (like pilates), meditation, and relaxation therapies accomplished through breathing exercise, muscle relaxation, or guided imagery.

While alternative therapies were once dismissed by licensed physicians in recent years it has rapidly received more acceptance in conventional Western medicine and has become increasingly commonplace for treatment of a large number health conditions.

National Center for Complementary and Alternative Medicine (NCCAM)

The National Center for Complementary and Alternative Medicine (NCCAM) researches alternative medical therapies and is an agency within the larger National Institutes of Health. The NCCAM research database allows users to search for medical research related to specific health conditions and alternative medicine at http://nccam.nih.gov/health/atoz.htm. To perform a search simply enter your keywords in the search box and select "Search" or use the index of health topics located on the same page.

Nutrition

Doctors have long recognized the association between good nutrition and good health. Nutrition is the science of foods and nutrients contained in food. Nutrients found in food are used by the body to support growth, provide energy, and maintain and support body tissue. Thus, the study of nutrition examines the relationship between diet and health, including the relationship between diet and disease. Examples of chronic health conditions commonly associated with nutrition include Cardiovascular Disease, Obesity, Type II Diabetes, Osteoporosis, and Hypertension.

National Institutes of Health Office of Dietary Supplements (ODS)

The National Institutes of Health Office of Dietary Supplements (ODS) is an office of the National Institutes of Health and provides users a searchable database containing bibliographic information about nutrition and health and disease. The database, called the International Bibliographic Information on Dietary Supplements, or IBIDS for short can be accessed free of charge at http://ods.od.nih.gov/Health_Information/IBIDS.aspx.

The IBIDS database is provided under a collaborative effort between the National Institutes of Health and the U.S. Department of Agriculture. Searching the database simply involves typing your search terms in the box and selecting "Search."

Biotechnology & Patents

Biotechnology is the application of technology to manufacture products that improve biological processes for the benefit of living organisms. In medicine, biotechnology is the basis for the development of pharmaceutical drugs, diagnostic and testing equipment, surgical implants, assisted living devices, and nearly every other tangible product that improves patient lives and outcomes.

A **patent** is a form of **intellectual property**. Intellectual property is distinct from tangible property and refers to creations of the mind. Just as physical property rights protect a person from encroachment on tangle items, intellectual property rights protect a person from encroachment of creations of the mind. Intellectual property is generally divided into two categories, industrial property and copyright. Most often copyright applies to artistic works, like song lyrics, music scores, poems, novels, artistic paintings, photographs, and sculptures. Industrial property includes trademarks, industrial design, and patents and generally apply to physical items that are of utility for human use. Industrial property includes the ideas, thought, and reason that form the basis of an invention and are commonly expressed in mathematical calculations, engineering design, and the manipulation and combination of chemical processes and properties.

Most biotechnological creations are protected by patents. Most often intellectual property rights are asserted to prohibit **another** party from using creations of the mind in their own profit-making ventures. In addition to patents and copyright, two other common types of intellectual property are trademark and trade secrets. It is important to remember that intellectual property rights do **not** imply ownership, but rather the right to control the commercialization of the ideas or expression in question.

Patents can be an excellent source of information about not only patented drugs and medical devices but about disease and health conditions in general. Since patents are organized in a uniform and consistent manner, the introduction or background section can provide an excellent review of current scientific literature about a disease and also detailed discussions about various health care topics.

While property rights to physical items establish exclusive ownership rights to property that can be seen and felt, intellectual property rights establish ownership rights to creations of the mind. Besides patents, copyright and trademarks are the most the common types of intellectual property. According the U.S. Patent and Trademark Office: "a patent is an intellectual property right granted by the Government of the United States of America to an inventor 'to exclude others from making, using, offering for sale, or selling the invention throughout the United States or importing the invention into the United States' for a limited time in exchange for public disclosure of the invention when the patent is granted." ("USPTO Glossary," n.d.)

Since patent applications are filed as long as five years before patent approval, these filings can give the researcher a glimpse into the future of the treatment, and sometimes even cures, for various diseases and health conditions.

While three types of patents can be granted, the two most common patents related to health care are **Utility Patents** and **Design Patents**. Utility patents protect inventions and discoveries of useful and new processes, machines, articles of manufacture, or "compositions of matter." As the name implies, design patents protect the drawings, charts, etc. that establish the shape and physical characteristics of an object to be manufactured. The third type of patent is the **Plant Patent** and is reserved for the discovery or invention of a new variety of "asexually" reproduced plant. Again, plant patents are uncommon in biotechnology.

Patent Information Online

The two most popular sources for patents granted in the United States are Google Patents https://www.google.com/patents and the U.S. Patent and Trademark Office by using either the quick search option http://patft.uspto.gov/netahtml/PTO/search-bool.html or the advanced search option http://patft.uspto.gov/netahtml/PTO/search-adv.htm.

The quick search option enables researchers to search up to two (2) research terms and also allows search results to be limited to specific fields or parts of the patent including applicant name and issue date.

Clinical Guidelines

As the name implies, a clinical guideline is a document that outlines the clinical management of a disease or health condition. In this regard, a clinical guideline can be viewed as a blueprint for the doctor and health care team to follow to diagnosis, manage, and treat specific health conditions in patients. Like any blueprint, however, the doctor must also incorporate her knowledge, experience, and best professional judgment and alter her application of a clinical guideline by taking into consideration the particular physical and emotional state of the patient, as well as the patients set of values and beliefs. Therefore, in practice the use of clinical guidelines by physicians is just that, a guideline used in conjunction with several other considerations to determine patient care.

Clinical guidelines generally cover every aspect of patient care, from diagnosis to treatment and prognosis and continuing care. The clinical guideline will typically also outline the risks and benefits of a course of action, as well as cost-effectiveness.

An important societal objective of clinical guidelines is to standardize medical care; thereby allowing patients regardless of income or socioeconomic status to receive the same high quality medical care.

Agency for Healthcare Research and Quality (AHRQ)

Clinical guidelines are generally collected and approved, and frequently written by a national health care agency. In the United States, the U.S. Agency for Healthcare Research and Quality (AHRQ) acts as the clearinghouse for clinical guidelines even though many are written by professional medical and doctor and associations. The AHRQ collection of guidelines can be accessed at http://www.guideline.gov/. Searching clinical guidelines at AHRQ is easy as the site uses similar syntax as a normal web search. Thus, to find a guideline for treating a specific disease simply enter your term in the search box. Likewise, to search for guidelines for conditions containing multiple words or phrases, enclose your terms in quotation marks. Finally, boolean searches can be performed using "and" or "or" between words and concepts of interest.

Drugs & Medications

Drugs are chemical substances that have a biological effect on humans and animals. Drugs are used by physicians to treat, cure, prevent, and even diagnose disease. Additionally, drugs can be used to enhance or improve mental or physical or well-being. Both prescription and over-the-counter drugs play several important roles in medicine. Drugs used to prevent disease are known as **Prophylactic Drugs**, drugs used to relieve symptoms are called **Palliative Drugs** and drugs used to cure disease are **Therapeutic Drugs**. Drugs for these purposes are also called medications or medicine, thus distinguishing them from drugs used for recreational or illicit purposes.

While all approved drugs have specific medicinal properties, most also have side effects. Side effects are secondary effects of medication that generally have no therapeutic value in the cure, treatment, or prevention of disease. Side effects can be both good and bad, but are most often the latter. One major challenge drug manufacturers face is developing medications that maximize the therapeutic effects of a drug while minimizing side effects. When prescribing medications or recommending over-the-counter alternatives, doctors consider both the "good" and the "bad" when determining the best course of medicinal treatment for patients.

Prescription and Over-the-Counter Drugs and Medications

The best single resource to research drugs and medications is the **Drug Information Portal** administered by the National Institutes of Health (NIH). Unlike a standard web database, a portal is a site that functions as a point of access to multiple search engines or databases on the Internet. The NIH Drug Information Portal simultaneously searches for summary and detailed information across a number of federal government drug databases. While the number of actual sources returned varies depending on the drug searched, each drug term entered will be searched in the following databases:

Databases Providing Summary Information:

- Drug information (MedlinePlusDrug)
-
    - http://www.nlm.nih.gov/medlineplus/druginformation.html
- Dietary supplements and herbs (MedlinePlusSupp)
-

  - http://www.nlm.nih.gov/medlineplus/druginfo/herb_All.html
* Consumer health information (MedlinePlusTopics)
*
  - http://www.nlm.nih.gov/medlineplus/
* HIV/AIDS treatment (AIDSinfo)
*
  - http://www.aidsinfo.nih.gov/
* Breastfeeding (LactMed)
*
  - http://toxnet.nlm.nih.gov/newtoxnet/lactmed.htm
* Drug-Induced Liver Injury (LiverTox)
*
  - http://livertox.nih.gov/
* Drug labels (DailyMed)
*
  - http://dailymed.nlm.nih.gov/
* Ingredients found in dietary supplements (Dietary Supplements Labels Database)
*
  - http://www.dsld.nlm.nih.gov/dsld/
* Clinical trials (ClinicalTrials.gov)
*
  - https://clinicaltrials.gov/
* Drug Identification with images (Pillbox beta)
*
  - http://pillbox.nlm.nih.gov/

Databases Providing Detailed Summary Information:
* Biological and physical data (HSDB)
*
  - http://toxnet.nlm.nih.gov/cgi-bin/sis/htmlgen?HSDB
* Scientific journals (Medline/PubMed)

-
  - http://www.ncbi.nlm.nih.gov/pubmed
- Toxicological journals (TOXLINE)
-
  - http://toxnet.nlm.nih.gov/cgi-bin/sis/htmlgen?TOXLINE
- Biological and chemical structures (PubChem)
-
  - https://pubchem.ncbi.nlm.nih.gov/
- Biological components of viruses (NIAID ChemDB)
-
  - http://chemdb.niaid.nih.gov/
- Toxicology and chemical components (ChemIDplus)
-
  - http://chem.sis.nlm.nih.gov/chemidplus/

Additional Drug Information Resources

- U.S. Food & Drug Administration (Drugs@FDA)
-
  - http://www.accessdata.fda.gov/scripts/cder/drugsatfda/
- U.S. Drug Enforcement Administration (DEA)
-
  - http://www.deadiversion.usdoj.gov/
- U.S. government search engine for all government resources (USA.gov)
-
  - http://www.usa.gov/

Information on more than 49,000 drugs and medications is included in the portal and drugs can be searched by either drug name or drug category (anticonvulsants, antidepressants, hallucinogens, etc.). The Drug Information portal is located at: http://druginfo.nlm.nih.gov/drugportal/drugportal.jsp

Books

Books can be an excellent source of medical information about Burning Mouth Syndrome. Typically, the best books can provide the researcher with both excellent background information and wide-ranging (but less in-depth) treatment about a health condition or disease. Books are best when you need a broad overview about a health condition, or you want to learn a "little about a lot" of topics associated with a disease or disorder. Books are also appropriate when you don't need timely or cutting-edge information about a health condition. In this regard, books are best for well-established health conditions, with a substantial and long-term history of general consensus regarding diagnosis, cause, treatment, and management protocols.

There are several reasons that books may be of limited utility for research purposes. First, the time between researching and writing a book to book publication and public availability can be a lengthy one. As such, for new health conditions, or those with evolving or ever-changing diagnostic standards or treatment protocols books may not be the best research option. Also, given the intense competition for readers, and space on the local bookstore shelves, books are necessarily broad-based to appeal to as many prospective readers as possible, and seldom address (or adequately address) obscure health conditions or narrow topics within a disease sufficiently.

While large retailers, like Amazon, Barnes and Noble, and WalMart may be excellent places to *purchase* books, they are not necessarily the best sources to *choose* which books contain the most authoritative and reliable information about Burning Mouth Syndrome, regardless of whether the book is a recent "best seller" or achieves positive reader reviews. Suffice to say, numerous media reports have documented the ease by which authors and publishers are able to artificially inflate book sales and accumulate glowing book buyer reviews.

National Library of Medicine's Bookshelf

The National Library of Medicine (NLM) Bookshelf provides anyone free access to book citations and other documents of interest for researching topics in health, medicine, and other life sciences. Bookshelf allows users to browse general topics or search for specific information about health conditions and disease in thousands of high-quality, well-researched books. Some books listed here even allow the researcher to read a portion or the entire contents of a book or document online.

To access Bookshelf, simply go to http://www.ncbi.nlm.nih.gov/books and begin your research by either browsing or searching for available titles. The interface is user friendly and allows the reader to browse by subjects including Health Care, Evidence-based Medicine, Health Policy, Comparative Effectiveness Research, and Public Health. Additional filters are also available to search by Book, Report, Collection, Documentation, or Database.

Below are a number of authoritative book and document titles related to Burning Mouth Syndrome.

Journals

Scholarly or academic health journals are different from the popular magazines you see in your supermarket or book store in a number of ways. Overall, while popular magazines are published to entertain a wide audience, academic health journals are written to advance the knowledge in a particular health related field. Other important differences between scholarly or academic journals and consumer magazines include:

1. Scholarly health journals publish **in-depth** articles by **experts** including **original** findings by the researcher who is also the article author. Popular magazines publish **general** information about someone else's findings.

2. Scholarly health journals take care to provide complete author **credentials** to demonstrate the author's subject-matter expertise. Popular magazine authors are almost **professional writers** with no subject matter expertise.

3. Scholarly health journals use **specialized terminologies** with very specific meanings. Popular magazine are taught to use only words and terms that a typical 7th grade reader can understand to make sure articles appeal to a broad readership.

4. Scholarly health journals are typically read only by other **scholars**, **researchers**, and **students** in the health care field. Popular magazines are read by the **general public**, most of whom will have no particular expertise, interest, or background in health care.

5. Scholarly health journals make prominent use of **graphs**, **tables**, and **charts**. Popular magazines include glossy **graphics** and **photographs**, along with significant **advertising**.

6. Scholarly health journal articles follow are very specific **format** and **layout**. Popular magazine format is generally **informal**.

7. Scholarly health journal articles include many carefully chosen **references**. Popular magazines seldom use references and instead use seemingly random **quotations** by experts and others.

8. Scholarly health journal articles are **peer-reviewed** by other subject-matter experts to ensure accuracy. Popular magazines are **edited** by editors with no subject-matter expertise.

The following section instructs you on how to find the most important journals related to Burning Mouth Syndrome and also lists the most important titles for further review.

MEDLINE Journals - The Abridged Index Medicus (AIM)

The National Institutes of Health (NIH), National Library of Medicine (NLM) MEDLINE and PubMed research databases currently provide anyone with internet access to citations for over 5,600 journal titles. The Abridged Index Medicus (AIM) was created to assist researchers by limiting the vast NLM holdings to a manageable number of important or "core" journals. AIM is provided by the NLM to "afford rapid access to selected biomedical journal literature of immediate interest to the practicing physician" and therefore, in the opinion of NLM researchers, represents the most important medical journals for the broadest numbers of physicians. AIM is available online as a subset of PubMed by limiting searches to "Core clinical journals." The complete current list of AIM core journals can be found by going to http://www.nlm.nih.gov/bsd/aim.html.

All MEDLINE Journals

Using PubMed, it is easy to find the journals related to the specific medical conditions, disorders, or issues important to you. Like any database, however, there are specific search strategies that will make retrieving information easier.

Current Journals

Due to the large number of journals currently indexed in MEDLINE, it is seldom feasible to print out the entire list. However, if you do want to view and save the entire updated list there are two primary methods.

For current titles indexed by MEDLINE go to the "NLM Catalog" at: http://www.ncbi.nlm.nih.gov/nlmcatalog and in the search box enter the term: **currentlyindexed** then click search.

A second method is to type **all [sb]** in the search box. Once the results appear go to the "**Journal subsets filter**" on the left sidebar of the page and "**More...**"

The selection will then expand as a pop-up box will display "**Journal subsets**". Make sure only the box entitled "**Currently indexed in MEDLINE**" is selected and go to the bottom of the popup and click the blue "**Show**" button.

While nothing appears to happen you will now see the "**Currently indexed in MEDLINE**" filter the Journal Subsets list on located on the sidebar. Click the "**x**" in the popup to close it and then click on "**Currently indexed in MEDLINE**" filter in the left sidebar. This will rerun the search and return all journals currently indexed in MEDLINE.

In 2014, this search returned 5,663 unique journal titles currently indexed in the NLM catalog.

To save a copy of the search results, find the hyperlink entitled "**Send to:**" located near the top of the search page and just left of the sidebar on the right. From there you can choose to send as an email, save to a temporary clipboard, or save as text document.

If ever you need to start over, you can delete all filters by simply clicking "**clear**" located just to the right of "**Journal subsets**" in the left sidebar.

Current and Previously Indexed Journals

For journals that were once indexed by MEDLINE but are no longer indexed **and** journals currently indexed the search protocol is almost identical to the search for **All Current Journals**, except for minor changes in the search term or filter, depending on which you method you use.

Again, go to the "NLM Catalog" at: http://www.ncbi.nlm.nih.gov/nlmcatalog and in the search box enter the term: **reportedmedline** then click search.

A second method is to type **all [sb]** in the search box and then click search. Once the results appear go to the "**Journal subsets filter**" on the left sidebar of the page and "**More...**"

The selection will then expand as a pop-up box and display "**Journal subsets**". This time make sure only the box entitled "**Journals currently or previously indexed in MEDLINE.**" is selected and go to the bottom of the popup and click the blue "**Show**" button.

Again, while nothing appears to happen you will now see that the **"Journals currently or previously indexed in MEDLINE"** filter is active in the Journal Subsets filter list. Click the close icon, marked as **"X"**, in the popup to close it and then click on **"Journals currently or previously indexed in MEDLINE"** filter in the left sidebar. This will rerun the search and return all journals both formerly and currently indexed in MEDLINE.

In 2014, this search returned 14,804 unique journal titles both currently and previously indexed in the NLM catalog.

To save a copy of the search results, find the hyperlink entitled **"Send to:"** located near the top of the page, and just left of the right sidebar. From there you can choose to send the complete list as an email, save to a temporary clipboard, or save as a text document.

If ever you need to start over, you can delete all filters by simply clicking **"clear"** located just to the right of **"Journal subsets"** in the left sidebar.

To find journals related to Burning Mouth Syndrome go to the NLM **Broad Subject Terms for Indexed Journals** web page at http://wwwcf.nlm.nih.gov/serials/journals/index.cfm. Arranged alphabetically, this is the MEDLINE catalog page for all journals related to specific diseases, disorders, and conditions and other medical issues. Simple select the letter [*correct letter here*] and scroll to and click Burning Mouth Syndrome and a list of relevant journals will display.

To save a copy of the search results, again find the hyperlink entitled **"Send to:"** located near the top of the page and just left of the right sidebar. From there you can choose to send as an email, save to a temporary clipboard, or save as text document.

Using Filters to Search

Given the enormous amount of information stored by the NLM, the use of database filters is important to narrow your search to only relevant information. In the previous section, the use of the **"Currently indexed in MEDLINE"** and **"Journals currently or previously indexed in MEDLINE"** were explained but there are several other useful filters to help focus your research.

Use the NLM **Catalog filters** to collect dental, consumer health, or other journal subset lists:

First, retrieve all items in the **NLM Catalog**

http://www.ncbi.nlm.nih.gov/nlmcatalog/ homepage and enter all [sb] in the search box.

In the Filters sidebar located on the Results page, click on **Currently indexed in MEDLINE**. If you require a different subset, instead of selecting **"Currently indexed in MEDLINE"**, click **"More"** and additional filtering options will display in a pop-up. The available filters allow you to construct subsets from the following journal categories:

- **Journals in electronic-only format**
- **Journals indexed from the electronic version**
- **Consumer Health journals**
- **Core clinical journals (AIM)**
- **Dental journals**
- **Index Medicus journals (IM)**
- **Nursing journals**
- **Additional subsets in the journal subset lists include:**
- **Referenced in NCBI DBs**
- **Only PubMed journals**
- **Currently indexed in MEDLINE**
- **Journals currently or previously indexed in MEDLINE**
- **PubMed Central journals**
- **PubMed Central forthcoming journals**

Check the box next to the filter you need and click the **"Show"** button. The selected filter will now be visible on the sidebar filter. Close the pop-up box and click the filter on the sidebar. This will re-run your search limiting the results to the filter you selected.

Journal Articles

In this last chapter we identified methods for finding the most important journals **titles** related to Burning Mouth Syndrome. This chapter expands on this information by identifying the best methods to search for **articles** in these journal titles and other academic health publications. During the course of your review, remember that unlike popular magazines academic journals are written and structured in a very standard and formal manner. While you may consider the format or structure bland and unappealing, remember the fundamental purpose of journal articles is to impart knowledge and communicate information and not to entertain. In this regard, it is this structured and nondescript presentation of information that lends itself particularly well to communicating important medical information.

Journal articles are a primary research resource. They are typically narrowly-focused and are the best literature resource for high quality and concentrated treatment of a topic. Scholarly articles are written by experts, incorporate complex data and statistics, and often times are used to present the most important and cutting-edge information about the recognition and treatment of disease and health conditions. Furthermore, scholarly journals are peer-reviewed meaning they are not only written by experts but are also carefully and critically reviewed by other experts before publication.

Academic and scholarly health journal articles are the best resources for very recent information about a health disease or disorder and for narrow topics within the larger context of a health condition.

Types of Research Articles

Most medical journal articles fall into one of two article categories: basic biomedical research or clinical research.

Biomedical research is the study of how living beings function. Human bodies are composed of smaller living systems that have their own unique life cycles. Similarly, disease has a life cycle and how that cycle functions in the human body is the subject of many research papers. Basic research in biomedical sciences may investigate the way basic protein sequences work in living things. Biomedical research can explain how cells appear, replicate, communicate, function, die, and then disappear. Biomedical research is important because the processes studied can effect disease or ensure good health. Biomedical research seeks to define biological processes and to understand learn how the body functions when disease is present and when disease is absent. Research leading to the understanding of these processes results in the development of drugs and other therapies that can disrupt disease mechanisms and restore the body to good health. Often, biomedical research use insect, fish, or animal test subjects in place of humans.

Clinical research is a the branch of medical science that explores the safety and effectiveness of medical devices, diagnostic tests, and drug and other medical treatments intended for human use. Clinical research can be subdivided into three different types. The first is **patient-oriented research**. Patient-oriented research is conducted with human subjects. Unlike Biomedical research, the scientists interact directly with the people involved in the study. A variety of reasons may be given to use patient-oriented research such as investigating human disease mechanisms, therapeutic interventions, clinical trials and/or development of new technologies. A second class of clinical research is **epidemiology**. "Epidemiology is the study of the distribution and determinants of health-related states or events (including disease), and the application of this study to the control of diseases and other health problems." ("Epidemiology," n.d.)

The final type of clinical research is **behavioral studies**. Behavioral studies focus on the actions, behaviors, and responses of individuals, groups, or species in its natural environment. The way a living being reacts to stimulation in regards to action and response is considered behavior. Behavior scientists studies are conducted on both humans and other animals and seek descriptions, generalizations, and explanations of behavior.

Clinical research can also be performed in the fields of physiology, pathophysiology, mental health and health services, education, and outcomes but are less common than the types of research discussed above.

The National Library of Medicine

This section focuses on the three most popular health-research databases, all administered by the National Institutes of Health (NIH), National Library of Medicine. These databases were chosen for several reasons. First, the NIH databases contain the most comprehensive and respected collection of academic and professional journal reference information available today. Second, the NIH databases are free to anyone with an Internet connection. While other excellent databases do exist, most simply "interface" with the NIH databases and can cost several hundreds, or even thousands of dollars a month to access.

The singular mission of the NIH is to perform original scientific biomedical and health research. As mentioned earlier, NIH researchers in the **Intramural Research Program (IRP)** perform in-house research and professionals in the **Extramural Research Program (ERP)** provide funding for research performed by scientists in academic institutions and other scientific research organizations. In 2013, 8,000 research grants were awarded funding out of nearly 50,000 applications received. Each year, approximately one-fourth of all scientific health research in the United States is fund by the NIH.

The NIH, National Library of Medicine (NLM) is the world's largest health research and biomedical library. Among its on-site holdings are more than 7 million medical-related books, journals, manuscripts, transcripts, and medical images. Perhaps even more impressive, is the NLM's online databases, search engine, and tools that allow scientists and the general public worldwide to access vital health-related information, including journal articles and data, and perform important medical research.

National Library of Medicine Databases

The three major information resources provided by the NLM are **MEDLINE, PubMed, and PubMed Central**.

MEDLINE

MEDLINE is comprised of scholary journal citations (including abstracts) for life science published in the U.S. and internationally. MEDLINE contains citations for approximately 5,400 biomedical journals published in the United States and worldwide. Coverage includes more than 21 million citations dating back to 1946. The MEDLINE database includes citations and abstracts in the fields of medicine, nursing, dentistry, veterinary medicine, health care systems and pre-clinical sciences to be offered through PubMed.

PubMed

PubMed consists of nearly 24 million citations for health science literature found in MEDLINE, books, and academic journals. Journal article citations link directly full-text articles and papers in PubMed Central and to publisher sites for articles not archived in PubMed Central. PubMed is free resource and available throughout the world.

PubMed Central

PubMed Central is a vast archive of medical and life science journal literature. Notably, all literature in PubMed Central is full-text meaning anyone can access the some of most important medical research conducted throughout the world.

PubMed Journal Citations

To begin using searching strategies outlined above enter your search term at

REFERENCES

Abraham, J., Gulley, J. L., & Allegra, C. J. (2010). *Bethesda handbook of clinical oncology*. Philadelphia, PA: Lippincott Williams & Wilkins.

Atlas of pathophysiology. (2010). Philadelphia: Wolters Kluwer Health/Lippincott Williams & Wilkins.

Beers, M. H., & Fletcher, A. J. (2004). *The Merck manual of medical information*. New York: Pocket Books.

Bratton, R. L. (2007). *Bratton's family medicine board review*. Philadelphia: Lippincott Williams & Wilkins.

Brown, L. J., & Miller, L. T. (2005). *Pediatrics*. Philadelphia: Lippincott Williams & Wilkins.

Cecil, R. L., Goldman, L., & Ausiello, D. A. (2008). *Cecil medicine*. Philadelphia: Saunders Elsevier.

Chabner, B., & Longo, D. L. (2011). *Cancer chemotherapy and biotherapy: Principles and practice*. Philadelphia: Wolters Kluwer Health/Lippincott Williams & Wilkins.

Colledge, N. R., Walker, B. R., Ralston, S., & Davidson, S. (2010). *Davidson's principles and practice of medicine*. Edinburgh: Churchill Livingstone/Elsevier.

Collier, J. A., Longmore, J. M., & Brinsden, M. (2006). *Oxford handbook of clinical specialties*. Oxford: Oxford University Press.

Collins, C. E., & DePetris, A. (2011). *A short course in medical terminology*. Baltimore, MD: Wolters Kluwer Health/Lippincott Williams & Wilkins.

Collins, J., & Stern, E. J. (2008). *Chest radiology: The essentials*. Philadelphia: Wolters Kluwer Health/Lippincott Williams & Wilkins.

Collins, R. D. (2008). *Differential diagnosis in primary care*. Philadelphia: Lippincott Williams & Wilkins.

Crabtree, T. D., Foley, E. F., & Sawyer, R. G. (2000). *General surgery*. Philadelphia: Lippincott William & Wilkins.

Dale, D. C. (2007). *ACP Medicine*. New York: WebMD.

Davidson, R. J. (2000). *Anxiety, depression, and emotion*. Oxford: Oxford University Press.

Diaz, S. E. (2006). *The little black book of emergency medicine*. Sudbury, MA: Jones and Bartlett.

Dictionary of Cancer Terms. (n.d.). Retrieved from http://cancergenome.nih.gov/Common/PopUps/popDefinition.aspx?id=CDR0000045022&version=Patient&language=English

Domino, F. J., & Baldor, R. A. (2012). *The 5-minute clinical consult 2012*. Philadelphia, PA: Wolters Kluwer Health/Lippincott Williams & Wilkins.

Dudek, R. W. (2010). *Genetics*. Baltimore, MD: Lippincott Williams & Wilkins.

Eichenbaum, H., & Cohen, N. J. (2004). *From conditioning to conscious recollection: Memory systems of the brain*. Oxford: Oxford University Press.

Epidemiology. (n.d.). Retrieved from http://www.who.int/topics/epidemiology/en/

Ferri, F. F. (2007). *Practical guide to the care of the medical patient*. Philadelphia: Mosby/Elsevier.

Ferri, F. F. (2008). *Ferri's clinical advisor 2008: Instant diagnosis and treatment*. St. Louis, MO: Elsevier Mosby.

Fischbach, F. T., & Dunning, M. B. (2009). *A manual of laboratory and diagnostic tests*. Philadelphia: Wolters Kluwer Health/Lippincott Williams & Wilkins.

Flynn, J. A., Choi, M. J., & Wooster, L. D. (2013). *Oxford American handbook of clinical medicine*. Oxford: Oxford University Press.

Goetz, C. G. (2007). *Textbook of clinical neurology*. Philadelphia: Saunders Elsevier.

Gonzales, R., & Kutner, J. S. (2007). *Current practice guidelines in primary care 2007*. New York: McGraw-Hill Medical.

Gorbach, S. L. (2001). *The 5 minute infectious diseases consult*. Philadelphia: Lippincott Williams & Wilkins.

Griffin, B. P., Rimmerman, C. M., & Topol, E. J. (2007). *The Cleveland Clinic cardiology board review*. Philadelphia: Lippincott Williams & Wilkins.

Handbook of diseases. (2004). Philadelphia: Lippincott Williams & Wilkins.

Harrison's principles of internal medicine. (2012). New York, N.Y.:

McGraw-Hill.

Hay, D. W. (2011). *The little black book of gastroenterology*. Sudbury, MA: Jones & Bartlett Learning.

Hay, W. W. (2007). *Current pediatric diagnosis & treatment*. New York: Lange Medical Books/McGraw-Hill, Medical Pub. Division.

Higgins, E. S., & George, M. S. (2007). *The neuroscience of clinical psychiatry: The pathophysiology of behavior and mental illness*. Philadelphia: Wolters Kluwer Health/Lippincott Williams & Wilkins.

Jonsen, A. R., Siegler, M., & Winslade, W. J. (2010). *Clinical ethics: A practical approach to ethical decisions in clinical medicine*. New York: McGraw-Hill Medical.

Karp, S. J., Morris, J., & Zaslau, S. (2008). *Blueprints surgery*. Philadelphia: Wolters Kluwer Health/Lippincott Williams & Wilkins.

Katz, D. L., & Friedman, R. S. (2008). *Nutrition in clinical practice: A comprehensive, evidence-based manual for the practitioner*. Philadelphia: Lippincott Williams & Wilkins.

Kumar, V., & Robbins, S. L. (2007). *Robbins basic pathology*. Philadelphia, PA: Saunders/Elsevier.

Kupfer, D. J. (2008). *Oxford American handbook of psychiatry*. Oxford: Oxford University Press.

Longmore, J. M., & Longmore, J. M. (2007). *Oxford handbook of clinical medicine*. Oxford: Oxford University Press.

Longo, D. L., & Harrison, T. R. (2012). *Harrison's principles of internal medicine*. New York: McGraw-Hill, Medical.

McLatchie, G. R., Borley, N. R., Chikwe, J., & McLatchie, G. R. (2007). *Oxford handbook of clinical surgery*. Oxford: Oxford University Press.

McPhee, S. J., & Hammer, G. D. (2010). *Pathophysiology of disease: An introduction to clinical medicine*. New York: McGraw-Hill Medical.

McPhee, S. J., & Papadakis, M. A. (2011). *Current medical diagnosis & treatment 2011*. New York: McGraw-Hill Medical.

Nicoll, D., McPhee, S. J., & Pignone, M. (2003). *Pocket guide to diagnostic tests*. New York: McGraw-Hill.

Olesen, J. (2006). *The headaches*. Philadelphia: Lippincott Williams & Wilkins.

Orient, J. M., & Sapira, J. D. (2005). *Sapira's art & science of bedside diagnosis*. Philadelphia: Lippincott Williams & Wilkins.

Phibbs, B. (2007). *The human heart: A basic guide to heart disease*. Philadelphia: Lippincott Williams & Wilkins.

Pocock, G., & Richards, C. D. (2006). *Human physiology: The basis of medicine*. Oxford: Oxford University Press.

Professional guide to signs & symptoms. (2007). Philadelphia: Lippincott Williams & Wilkins.

Rakel, R. E. (2007). *Textbook of family medicine*. Philadelphia: Saunders/Elsevier.

Robbins, S. L., Kumar, V., & Cotran, R. S. (2010). *Robbins and Cotran pathologic basis of disease*. Philadelphia, PA: Saunders/Elsevier.

Sackett, D. L., Rosenberg, W. M., Gray, J. A., Haynes, R. B., & Richardson, W. S. (1996). Evidence based medicine: What it is and what it isn't. *Bmj, 312*(7023), 71-72. doi:10.1136/bmj.312.7023.71

Schein, M., & Rogers, P. N. (2005). *Schein's common sense emergency abdominal surgery*. Berlin: Springer.

Schrier, R. W. (2007). *The internal medicine casebook: Real patients, real answers*. Philadelphia: Lippincott Williams & Wilkins.

Shader, R. I. (2003). *Manual of psychiatric therapeutics*. Philadelphia: Lippincott Williams & Wilkins.

Snell, R. S., & Snell, R. S. (2008). *Clinical anatomy by regions*. Philadelphia: Lippincott Williams & Wilkins.

Thomas, J., & Monaghan, T. (n.d.). *Oxford handbook of clinical examination and practical skills*.

Tintinalli, J. E., & Stapczynski, J. S. (2011). *Tintinalli's emergency medicine: A comprehensive study guide*. New York: McGraw-Hill.

Topol, E. J., & Califf, R. M. (2007). *Textbook of cardiovascular medicine*. Philadelphia: Lippincott Williams & Wilkins.

Tulving, E., & Craik, F. I. (2000). *The Oxford handbook of memory*. Oxford: Oxford University Press.

USPTO Glossary. (n.d.). Retrieved from
http://www.uspto.gov/main/glossary/

Warrell, D. A. (2003). *Oxford textbook of medicine*. Oxford: Oxford
University Press.

Wasson, J. (2009). *The common symptom guide: A guide to the evaluation of
common adult and pediatric symptoms*. New York: McGraw Hill Medical.

Westover, M. B., Choi, E., & Awad, K. M. (2010). *Pocket neurology*.
Philadelphia: Wolters Kluwer Health/Lippincott Williams & Wilkins.

Zuber, T. J., & Mayeaux, E. J. (2004). *Atlas of primary care procedures*.
Philadelphia: Lippincott Williams & Wilkins.